THE MEDICAL STUDENT'S GUIDE

I0390699

"A SHINING LIGHT ILLUMINATING THE PATH ON YOUR JOURNEY TO GET A MEDICAL DEGREE"

HENRY EGBUCHIEM BSc,M.D

For more about the book please visit:

henryegbuchiem.blogspot.com/2016/10/about-book-medical-students-guide.html

<u>DEDICATION</u>

This book is fondly dedicated to my parents (who continuously taught me the importance of hard work) and all those nursing the intent of becoming medical doctors.

TABLE OF CONTENTS

INTRODUCTION

Getting a medical degree is pretty much like embarking on a journey; agreeably, it may be a somewhat difficult journey to take because, even while you are quite abreast of the outcome of the journey and what you intend accomplishing at its end (Your MD!), you are often oblivious to the twist, turns and indeed, lurking ghosts ahead. Of course, there are those tales (some true and others false) that attempt to paint what is usually an unclear picture of what medical school is really like, but it is my opinion that these distorted tales are not only misleading but end up making the journey of obtaining a medical degree, less bearable.

It is in regard to this, that I write this book. With the stoic belief that it would serve not only as a simple manual but also as a precious guide for medical students all around the world as they embark on this uncertain journey. I hope, amidst all odds, that with this book, they'll be able to maneuver through the numerous challenges they'll come across and be equipped with relevant information that would both guide and illuminate their paths on this sacred sojourn.

WHO IS THIS BOOK FOR?

First and foremost, this book is designed for anyone that is interested in starting a medical career. Especially those that are just fresh out of high school and are in search of answers to their nagging questions concerning being a medical student or studying medicine. Or perhaps for those that aren't quite satisfied with the response they have gotten to the questions they once asked. I believe that with the wealth of information presented in this book, these needs would be met and all questions would be answered.

Secondly, this book can be used by those already in medical school who are presently experiencing the all-too-familiar low points, characterized by mental fatigue and depression that stem from memorizing and learning the vast amount of data befitting for a medical student or those that have had their belief in their will power and innate abilities crushed by the hurdles of medical school to the point that they feel it is practically impossible for them to continue studying medicine. Interestingly, if this looks like you, I want to say, "Don't fret!" Since embedded clearly in the passages of this book are a wealth of experience and sound advice that will undoubtedly help you overcome any challenge you seem to be facing, be it the meager problem of improper time management to the cumbersome task of determining your appropriate study habit, in no time I'm confident you'll get a hang of it and your medical journey would soon feel like a pleasant walk in a park!

In addition, if you are only interested in knowing the inner workings of the world of medicine and how each subject integrates with one another, this then is most definitely an indispensable tool for you because I am poised to explaining major concepts and key ideas that every medical practitioner should know. Allow me to state at this point, that although I don't intend writing a medical textbook, I am sure that this book can easily serve as a guide. In other words, before you read that cumbersome chapter with over a hundred pages from your regular textbook, you may use this material to have a generalized view of what you are expected to know and to ensure that proper emphasis is placed on the most relevant information.

Together as we start this journey (which is perhaps the most important journey you'll ever embark on) I'll try to expose the basic hurdles or challenges that you'll sooner than latter face and I promise to proffer meaningful solutions to these challenges so that you won't be caught unawares as they eventually come your way.

Just sit back and enjoy the ride!

CHAPTER ONE
THE BEGINNING!

THE IMPORTANCE AND PLACE OF MEDICINE IN OUR SOCIETY
Just before we commence on our journey, I will like to take you on a cursory look at what I consider to be the backbone of medicine. Or perhaps let's just say I'm setting the stage for what this book is supposed to be about!

Someone once defined medicine as "the science of the art of healing". In my opinion, this definition truly embodies what the principle of the study of medicine propagates. Amidst all the scientific and medical jargon, it is quite easy for someone to forget that perhaps medicine can and should also be viewed as an art. Yes, I said it, an art! One that encompasses an array of varied health care practices and customs that have been passed down from generations. Indeed, just like we learn a folklore or recipes, some practices in medicine have been transferred from one generation to another either through observation or apprenticeship, in form of songs, and in most recent times, scientific writings. Whether this is formal or not, the bottom line remains the same. Information is passed down to subsequent generations in a particular way that is both respected and accepted to people of a particular era.

As an art, medicine utilizes several principles that are resourceful in the healing of an individual patient. These principles though are not sacrosanct, because different fields in medicine often adopt variations that stem from a logical perspective. But it is important to realize that in other to come up with relevant conclusions which are reproducible in any part of the world, a set of rules and regulation must be adhered to. This is as true in any scientific endeavor as it is in medicine.

HENCE THE MAXIM THAT IS PERHAPS MOST OFTEN UPHELD AND EMPLOYED IN CLINICAL MEDICINE IRRESPECTIVE OF THE VARIOUS FIELDS, TO COME UP WITH DIAGNOSIS AND TREATMENT OF DISEASES IS EXPLAINED AS FOLLOWS:

I)   HISTORY TAKING

This includes asking the patient different questions concerning not only his disorder but also about his life, family background etc. You will be amazed to find out that with experience and proper history taking, most physicians manage to make an accurate diagnosis. This, of course, is an admirable trait that every single physician should strive for as it not only reduces the burden or cost of running expensive tests but it obliterates the unnecessary wasting of time. However, in some cases, patients aren't able to give comprehensive answers; such is usually experienced in pediatrics or geriatric practice. Nevertheless, one could always depend on the testimonies of parents, relatives or older siblings. In order to ensure that an excellent job is done for this part of the diagnosis and that no information is left unasked, we can further subdivide this section into the following.

A)   A collection of general information of a patient commonly called biodata. This includes their names, age or date of birth, marital status etc.

B)   Asking the patient about their chief complaints. This is often considered to be the most pressing complaints that bring the patient to the doctor. It is beneficial to document this part in the patient's own words and ensure that exact descriptions are made for every complaint. For example, if a patient says "my belly hurt", you should ask more questions in order to localize the pain, determine what type of pain it is (dull sharp, stabbing etc.), when the pain started, is the pain related to food intake and if taking a particular position reduces the intensity of the pain.

C)   Asking about the history of the disease. This is also called **ANAMNESIS MORBI**. Again, here we try to determine when the disease started. If it (the disease)had an acute, sub-acute or chronic course. We also consider what treatment or medications patients received and their effects on the disease. Since most diseases occur in form of syndromes and semiotic entities, an adequate understanding of the start and course of a presenting disease can be helpful in creating a differential diagnosis and determining the outcome of the disease.

D)   Asking about life history. This is also known as **ANAMNESIS VITAE**. This part varies from one specialty to another as emphases are in life's history that is relevant to the discrete pathology. However, certain information is a must here irrespective of the specialty, such as the presence of allergies to drugs, food etc., the contact of an infectious person in the last two week, history of vaccinations, social strata and standard of living, genealogical history and so on. It is noteworthy that in recent times, the concept of past medical history has been included in the process of obtaining a comprehensive picture of the patient's illness. Here you want to know if the patient has a chronic condition such as sickle cell disease, asthma, hypertension, diabetes mellitus, and epilepsy or if they have ever received a blood transfusion in the past or undergone surgical procedures.

II)   PHYSICAL EXAMINATION.

This entails the evaluation of the patient as a whole being with considerations of different systems (i.e. the respiratory, digestive cardiovascular, genital, neurological etc.).It is important that all systems are adequately evaluated, as this is beneficial in exposing otherwise hidden disorders or co-morbid conditions. Every physical examination should start by inspection; you'll be amazed at what you'll discover if you only take the time to observe your patients. Also, for this part of the patients' care, the doctors' hands can serve as valuable tools! Physicians can make a diagnosis by the age old skill of palpation and percussion. Different organs can be palpated and percussed to determined their size, shape, and consistency. This skill if properly perfected can be utilized in areas where there isn't equipment for making detailed instrumental viewing of internal structures or in an emergency setting. Finally, materials like a stethoscope, sphygmomanometer, and penlight are all important pocket contents that can be used in the physical examination to make an appropriate and complete diagnosis.

Having completed the physical examination one is often lead to a temporary conclusion often referred to as the preliminary diagnosis. After which a series of confirmatory test are ordered. This leads to the next part of the care of the patient.

A useful mnemonic that has helped many physicians in this aspect is the **IPPA** system, which stands for inspection, percussion, palpation and auscultation respectively. You will do well to use this scheme in your physical examination of patients.

III)   PLAN OF LABORATORY OR INSTRUMENTAL DIAGNOSIS

There are different protocols for different diseases. However, the usual hierarchy is to start from blood work with the determination of complete blood counts and biochemical compositions of the blood. Then imaging studies are done; this could range from the use of routine to contrast x-rays, computer tomography and MRI in internal organs pathologies to the collection of biopsies and use of different histochemical stains to visualize different pathologies in light or electron microscopes.

IV)   TREATMENT PLAN

For treatment, the following scheme can be used:

a)   Non-medical treatment

This includes setting a regimen (i.e. what you'll have the patient do, such as bed rest, physical activity etc.), Diet (here, you place the patient on a particular diet that is going to reduce exacerbation of his pathology or perhaps give little influence on his disease).

b)   The medical Therapy

This can be subdivided into the following:

•   Supportive medical therapy

•   Symptomatic medical therapy

•   Etiological medical therapy

•   Pathogenetic medical therapy

In my experience, thinking in this manner has helped in covering all aspects of patients' medication management.

V)   Epicrisis

Most times after treatment, the medical practitioner is expected to come up with a summary of events that transpired during the course of caring for the patient. This summary is called the epicrisis. Although some may consider this pointless and over-simplistic or further argue that there is no need since the patient is already getting better, I beg to differ; I believe that if properly adhered to, caring and managing patients wouldn't be so cumbersome. Especially with the epicrisis in mind, one can easily determine at what level of the patients' care one is and then make educated guesses of the outcome of therapy and the eventual prognosis of the disease.

From our discussion, we may conclude that as a scientific study, medicine has come a long way. If we take into cognizance the prehistoric periods where medicine was characterized as a mere herbalist and ritualistic arts by a priest, shamans or medicine men (as they were often called!), we definitely would readily appreciate the point we are today.

Of course, it's no news that the inputs from those past glorious eras have enormously influenced the way we practice medicine today, therefore it is important for us to not only recognize the talented few of the past but also celebrate them for their instrumental work to the development experienced in medicine.

The Egyptian Imhotep, who lived in the third millennium BC is considered to be the first physician in history to have his name recorded. However, the title of the father of medicine is bestowed on the Greek physician Hippocrates. This is because his contributions to medicine cannot be overemphasized. Apart from laying down the foundation for what is referred to as the rational approach in medicine (in respect to the Hippocratic Oath), he succeeded in classifying diseases into different clinical forms. He is even credited to have used the terms acute, chronic, epidemic, and endemic, exacerbation, relapse, crises, convalescence, and paroxysm. All of which are still in use, today.

Also, Galen, a fellow Greek physician ,that has the accolade as one of the greatest surgeons that have ever lived. Even in ancient time without the sophistication of modern equipment, he managed to conduct an operation on delicate human structures such as the eyes and brain.

Just like most other scientific fields, the development of medicine is closely related to History and certain historical events often interfered with the developmental course of science. It is recorded that after the fall of the Western Roman Empire and the onset of the middle ages, the Greek traditions and their practice of medicine experienced a gleam decline especially in Western Europe, however, it continued to blossom in the Byzantine (Eastern) Roman Empire. It is believed that sometime after 750 CE the works of Hippocrates and Galen were translated into Arabic, and Islamic physicians were engaged in several significant medical researchers. These included men like

Avicenna, Polymath, and others. The physician Avicenna is believed to have written the manuscript "the cannon of medicine".

During this era, the earliest forms of public hospitals were created in the form of Islamic Bimaristan Hospitals.

In the 14/15th centuries, the advent of the Black Death heralded a shift in the traditionally established way medicine was practiced. This meant that people no longer dogmatically believed ideas or concepts just because it was propagated by some prominent figure. Hence physicians like andrease vasalius were able to disprove some old erroneous theories. As a matter of fact, Andrease vasalius is believed to have written one of the most influential books on Anatomy "De Humani Coporis Fabrica"

Other notable discoveries in later periods include works of Antonie Van Leeuwenhoek who in 1676 enacted the scientific field of microbiology as he observed microscopically the structure of bacteria and other microorganisms. William Harvey described the circulatory system and Pierre Fauchard started the practice of dentistry.

The 18-19th centuries saw tremendous developments in modern research based medicine and a host of prominent physicians in different parts of the world can be recognized for their ground breaking works.

Today the greatest influence in medicine is going to be seen by those proponents that purport evidence-based medicine; this is a process where through systematic reviews and Meta-analysis, protocols and perhaps algorithms for the management of patients and practice of medicine are drawn.

The place of medicine in the modern world can indeed be explained by the Hippocratic Oath. Although many authors would rather have this oath tucked away in a corner at the ends of their books, I have decided to go against the crowd and do the exact opposite. I consider having the Hippocratic Oath at the end of the book a misnomer because if the oath does represent rules and regulations that guide a physician, isn't it more beneficial to have it in the beginning so that everyone can be abreast of the content. Most certainly anyone that goes through the Oath is bound to discover that its author had a proper understanding of what medicine should be and its place in the society.

THIS IS THE MODERN HIPPOCRATIC OATH

I swear in the presence of the almighty and before my family, my teachers and my peers that according to my ability and judgment I will keep this Oath and its stipulation.

To reckon all who have taught me this art equally dear to me as my parents in the same spirit and dedication to impart knowledge of the art of medicine to others. I will continue with diligence to keep abreast of the advances in medicine. I will teach without exception all who seek my ministration so long as the treatment of others is not compromised thereby, and I will seek the counsel of particularly skilled physician where indicated for the benefit of my patient

I will follow that method of treatment which according to my ability and judgment I consider for the benefit of my patients and abstain from whatever is harmful or mischievous. I will neither prescribe nor administer a lethal dose of medicine to any patient even if asked nor counsel any such thing nor perform the utmost disrespect for every human life from fertilization to natural death and reject abortion that deliberately takes a unique human life.

With purity, holiness and beneficence, I will pass my life and practice my art. Except for the prudent correction of an imminent danger, I will neither treat any patient nor carry out any research on a human being without the valid informed consent of the subject or appropriate legal protector thereof. Understanding that research must have its purpose the furtherance of the health of that individual into whatever patient setting I enter. I will go for the benefit of the sick and abstain from every voluntary act of mischief or corruption and further from the seduction of any patient.

Whatever in connection with my professional practice or not in connection with it I may see or hear in the lives of my patients which I ought not be spoken abroad, I will not divulge reckoning that all such should be kept secret.

While I continue to keep this oath unviolated, may it be granted to me to enjoy life and the practice of the art and science of medicine with the blessing of the almighty and respected by my peers and society, but should I trespass and violate this oath may the reverse be my lot.

WHY DO WE NEED THIS CHAPTER?

I would not be surprised if you have already asked yourself this question. Well, let me out rightly say that this chapter was included so that we may all come to appreciate the marvellous work that has already being done by great men in the forming of the field of medicine, without whom the study of medicine as a medical science would not be possible. I want you to reflect on what you have just read, ponder on every era and the different contributions made, small and great, erroneous and accurate.

Also by the end of this chapter I want your world view to change, in order words, I love for you to begin to see medicine in a new light. In case you haven't noticed, you are joining a "brotherhood" of great men like Hippocrates, Imhotep, and others! Therefore, you should be extremely proud of yourself and the journey you have embarked on. You need to start treating yourself with uttermost respect and comport yourself as an honorable member of your society.

To a large extent, you will be entrusted with perhaps what is arguably the most important task in the world, "the care for the human life". In other words, you will be saddled with the responsibility of restoring health and preserving human life. To the rich and poor, king or peasants you will be considered a healer, people of all races and gender will put their trust in you and hope that you come up with answers that would alleviate their pain and sufferings.

 As elucidated by the world health organization, "health is a state of complete physical, mental and social well-being of an individual" and as a physician, you are to ensure that all these components of a patient's health are satisfied to ensure that they have good health.

"Every man is a volume if you know how to read him"

William Ellery Channing

This is to say that you are not just treating or managing a discrete disorder rather you are in control of a human life, someone with fears, feelings, hopes, dreams, aspirations and etc. and as such, for every patient of yours, you are expected to give your all. This can be in form of spending extra hours after the stipulated working periods, away from love ones and family, or waking up early in the middle of the night to go attend to a patient in need, or making the uttermost sacrifice for a research paper that when published can change the course of treatment for millions.

Even if while ensconced on your sofa reading this book you are probably thinking that this is a long shot from what you think of yourself, I want to tell you that you are wrong! In medicine, you are only required to take baby steps. Endeavor to do your best at all times and like in a relay race it won't be difficult for someone else to take up the baton from you and finish the race in grand style. But you should always remember that no matter how minuscule your contribution may seem, the little you added is instrumental to making the race the grand success that it turned out to be.

Interestingly, if you work hard enough, men will someday write and albeit, read about you and your commitment to the development of medicine. Just like we read today about the great men of old who have contributed immensely to medicine, men that devoted their time and indeed their lives so that we may have a proper understanding of how the human body functions and its complicated structure I am convinced that one day people would come to write and read about you too.

"Hold fast to your dreams for if dreams die, life is a broken winged bird that cannot fly"

Lanston Hughes

CHAPTER TWO

WHY EMBARK ON THIS JOURNEY?

Over the years, I have asked some of my colleagues and teachers this very question, and I am often fascinated by the response I get from them. Some say that the reason they came into medicine is simply for the sake of humanity and because of their compassion, they want to help people. While others chide that they are in medicine for the fame, prestige, and wealth it affords. Also, I have learnt from a handful that they only stumbled into medicine because their parents who happened to doctors instructed them to follow the family's professional path.

Personally, I think that no one answer is sacrosanct. For me, my medical career journey started because I wanted to make an impact on my generation. I believed (and still do) that I have something good to offer the world and medicine is perhaps one of the ways I can easily and truly express myself.

In a more serious note, if by now you have not yet answered the important question of why you are embarking on this journey, I suggest you take moment and do so right now! Try to come up with an honest answer to the question, because as it turns out, if you really can't think of a good reason to be on this journey, I strongly suggest that you quit now. Since this is not a journey that you would want to take lightly.

"An average person with average talent, ambition and education, can outstrip the most brilliant genius in our society, if that person has clear, focused Goals"
-- Brian Tracy

In the following paragraphs, I will try to explain the importance of knowing your motivation and the primary reason for being in medicine. Sometimes while on this journey, your resolve to continue would be tested and all that you have left might be the stoic reason of why you started in the first place! In addition, most of the decisions you make as a physician concerning your career are very much hinged directly or indirectly on why you decided to study medicine. For example, if one is in medicine for the fame, prestige and wealth, there is the tendency to sway towards the more financially gratifying fields in medicine. It also means that being a general practice doctor isn't good enough and there's need to be further educated and obtain some form of specialization or consultancy that would add up to extra and/or more pay. This, of course, requires time and finances, both of which should be seriously considered!

In addition, we may find that in those who are in medicine because the urge to save lives and help others far overshadows that of financial gratification or wealth, there is a compelling force to do it on a large scale. Hence joining organizations like Doctors without border, the Red Cross or volunteering to disaster or war zones is something that they may easily consider without second guessing themselves or harboring second thoughts.

Whatever the case may be, it's crystal clear that the very reasons why you decided to become a doctor may very well affect most if not almost all the decisions you will ever make. In other words, the reasons are, metaphorically speaking, "the wells in which you draw the basis of the value system".

"If you can imagine it, you can achieve it. If you can dream it, you can become it"

William Arthur Ward

In a challenging world like one in which we find ourselves now, it's expedient that we do all in our power to be abreast of the numerous advancement around us. From the day to day discoveries and better methods or protocol of patients' management, as good physicians we should be aware of these developments and understand both their advantages and shortcoming so that we are able to adequately inform and educate our patients. However, the resolve to continue on this quest can only come if you are aware of what you're true motivations are.

With the steady rise in the growth of the population of the world, it is understandable that there is an urgent need for more doctors. And no matter how competitive or challenging the tasks of being one are, there are certain standards and qualities expected from every aspiring or practicing doctor. Some of which we have already dealt with in the previous chapter and others that we would mention in subsequent ones.

Importantly, the main aim of this chapter is to encourage you to have a mission statement, the foundation on which you may build a solid medical career. Even if you are just starting out or perhaps you are already in and currently stuck in one of the potholes that are scattered on the road to a medical degree, the bottom line is you need a mission statement to know where you are headed so that you are constantly reminded of why you so badly want to become a doctor.

"There are doctors and there are doctors" this happen to be a famous quote for one of my university professors. He often said this to encourage us to be the best we could individually ever be. And according to him, only those that are determined to go the extra mile get distinguished and celebrated as a doctor of doctors! Yes, the challenges are humongous, the journey bleak, but can it be done? The answer is yes! It can be done, and it has been done time and again. Most importantly, it can and should be done well. One of my inspirations for writing this book is not only to tell

you that it's possible but rather to also teach you how to do it well.

> *"Believe in yourself and there will come a day when others will have no choice but to believe with you"*
> **Cynthia Kersey**

Undoubtedly, a sure way to getting it right is simply by having a personalized mission statement stipulating why you are in medicine, so that when the challenges come to your Way(as they often do!) you will know where to turn.

Before we move on to the next chapter I have a little exercise for you and I strongly suggest that you do it before going on.

To do

a) Get a plain sheet of paper and a pen

b) Write out clearly in bold text the reasons why you want to be a medical doctor

c) Make several copies of the note

d) Place them in places where you can easily reach, preferably stick one on your mirror, your bed side wall or reading table.

e) When you wake up in the morning for the next four weeks I want you to read the note out load to yourself several times with great conviction.

f) You may decide to leave the note in place throughout your stay in medical school as a constant reminder or tell friends and family about it to ensure that they are aware of your aspirations and goals so that they can help you in reaching them.

CHAPTER THREE

THE THINGS YOU REQUIRE FOR THE JOURNEY

In this chapter, I would try to inform you about the things that you are to put in your luggage as we commence on this journey. Taking into consideration that there is a tendency to have a poorly packed bag filled with junk and other frivolous items that are not needed in your quest for a medical degree I promised to do all in my power to intimate you on the essentials that would not only make your backpack lighter but also filled with less nonsense!

It's one thing to have all the urge and motivation in the world for this journey but it's another to possess the essential components that can make the voyage a smooth sailing one. If there is one thing I hope to achieve at the end of this chapter and indeed this book, it is to teach you how you can meander through the bends and turns of obtaining a medical degree without much stress or hassle.

I will be listing twelve points here and at the end I want you to check them off your list to ensure that you have them before we start the journey. The points are:

1)   A SOUND MIND

This is perhaps the most important point to be made here. To become a medical doctor or to work as one, a sound mind is most definitely an indispensable tool or an unrivaled prerequisite. You need a sound mind to both comprehend the cumbersome workload of medical school and logically sail through the perilous storms that lay ahead of you till you retire.

As a medical student, you will be faced with people from different works of life, professors, nurses, patients and fellow students all of whom may not totally be sympathetic to your learning pace. And as such, you will be saddled with the task of relating with every one of them in a courteous and civilized manner even when they behave unruly to you. This can be debilitating because most often, not only do you need these individuals, especially if they are your teachers, but your final grade may hinge on their report concerning you. Therefore in dealings with them, you may need to show restraint and continuous evidence of a sound mind.

Personally, one of the biggest lessons I learnt while in medical school is that your teachers are always correct, even when they seem wrong! Being a very inquisitive student I often asked a lot of questions and although a handful of my teachers never had problems with this as I advanced through medical school I soon discovered that some others didn't quite fancy me asking too many questions.

I can't really tell if they felt challenged or worked up but I soon learnt the hard way to know those that are tolerant and those that aren't. However, I should say that when I look back at it, I conjecture that it was mostly young teachers and doctors that took offense with my questions, whereas the old professors often encouraged me and even considered my "question asking times" beneficial.

Not long after I learnt my lesson I decided to be more tactful. I knew if I wasn't subservient the young lectures may be threatened so if I suspected that I had a tutor that would be offended by my questions, I tried never to ask them questions publicly and if I didn't agree with what they say about a concept or phenomenon, I privately disagree with them respectfully, in the process stating the source of where I got my information and expressing it as my "confusion". Since I discovered that if I called it my confusion, they were less likely to be antagonistic and most times feel better trying to help me solve my confusion.

Of course, we can all agree that if I was not tactful and sound in my judgment of individuals, I would end up not being in good terms with my teachers and I would find it difficult learning anything from them as they would be unwilling to associate with me or teach me anything.

Undoubtedly, it takes a sound mind to thread the fine line that lies between learning and being at peace with ones teachers, colleagues, patients etc. learning medicine is best done in the form of apprenticeship, in other words, to teach someone the art of medicine you have to be willing and able to nurture them, to lovingly point out their mistakes respectfully and encourage them to be better. This can be a very difficult task, and as we see most often, instructors take out their frustrations on the shortcomings of their students, thereby hampering the learning process and creating an atmosphere inadequate for proper learning. Being equipped with a sound mind can help both students and teachers alike create a conducive learning environment that truly bothers on mutual respect, tolerance and the understanding required to expedite the whole schooling experience.

In addition, having a sound mind includes portraying a dynamic individual spiritual component. To face the trials in this journey you need to believe in something, be it God, mere luck, fate whatever you want to call it! You just can't go through medical school without the realization of the importance of life and the helplessness of man, especially as you are taught to create an illusion of hope embedded in the cloak of logical thinking and reasoning.

"The real winners in life are the people who look at every situation with an expectation that they can make it work or make it better."
Barbara Pletcher

So many times you may write examinations and be unsure of their outcome- then, only your faith or belief can sustain and grant you succor. As a Christian, my faith is in God and in the promises in his word. I turn to this when I am faced with the nefarious trials in medicine, whether this is dealing with a difficult teacher or waiting for the result of an examination that felt pretty difficult, his love and promises have always come through for me and I am always victorious.

II)   RECOGNISE THAT YOU WILL MAKE MISTAKES

Interestingly in this day and age, where most doctors consider themselves to be Gods and erroneously assume that they are immune to making mistakes. This is wrong! As a medical student and doctor, the best and perhaps most valuable knowledge you can add to those that you get from studying your "big textbooks" is that you can and will definitely make mistakes. Importantly, like I often say to students, if you want to make mistakes it is better to make them while you are still a student. As a matter of fact, it is your right to make mistakes isn't that why we have exams? So that we can see the mistakes you make, correct them before you are given a degree and tossed into the real world without supervision and guidance.

"It is better to have enough ideas for some of them to be wrong, than to be always right by having no ideas at all."

Edward de Bono

From my experience, I learned that the questions I failed as a student and the mistakes that followed often left me with a strong emotional link; therefore I was less likely to repeat the same mistakes again.

Also in class, I never hesitated to say I didn't understand something when I didn't! funny enough, it often turned out that more than half of the class were as confused as me but happen to be reluctant to speak up and state that they don't understand because to them, it just was not cool not to know.

Believe me, when I say this, in your medical journey, you are to hold yourself responsible for what you learn and how you manage to learn it. It is a personal struggle regardless of the fact that you may have classmates or colleagues. Understand that you cannot all grasp information at the same pace, some would learn faster than others. So you should determine what pace is best suited for you and endeavor to have the class structured around your learning pace and abilities. Especially when others are too busy trying not to make mistakes or simply playing God! You should be the one to remind them that we are all but mere mortals and as such bound to make mistakes.

The fear of not wanting to make mistakes or being viewed as being dumb force some students not to seek help from other students. This is one big pitfall because in medicine about ninety percent of what you know, you read or learn on your own and only about ten percent is what is given by your tutor. And of the ninety percent, you learn by yourself you will come to discover that more than half of that knowledge stems from what you hear, learn and get from fellow students and colleagues. So is it not wise then to suck it up and to meet that student and colleague for help? Medicine is one of those courses that you just can't make it all on your own accord. You need people to help you build on what you already know, make positive re-enforcement and help clarify gray areas. Truly there are some smart and gifted ones amongst us that are capable of learning complex material at the speed of light. As an advice I say, meet these ones, beg them if you may, just don't let them go until you have learnt that concept you find so difficult. Who knows, what you get from them may end up saving a life someday.

"Things don't go wrong and break your heart so you can become bitter and give up. They happen to break you down and build you up so you can be all that you were intended to be.
Charles "Tremendous" Jones

III)   YOU NEED GOOD HEALTH

I would start this point by stating something one of my female professors says; you are a doctor first and foremost for yourself, for your family, then for your patients. In trying to teach us the importance of good health as a doctor she admonishes us to be doctors first for ourselves. Seriously speaking, I cannot think of any patient that would want to visit a doctor who is himself sick!

So you should be "well" at all times. As you embark on this journey one thing you want for yourself is good health. You should flee from any activity that would and can hamper your health. This includes taking unnecessary risks like drunk driving, unprotected intercourse, ill protective clothing in winter, use of illicit drugs, improper protection during patient care (just to mention a few!)

You should learn to take charge of your health and adhere to the advice that you most probably give your patients. For instance, how can you tell or convince your patients to stop smoking when you both only just shared a stick of cigarette before the start of the interview?

No matter how good a physician you are if you don't have good health it would be practically difficult for you fully achieve your potential in managing patients. So in conclusion, I want to state that having a good health starts with watching and indeed diligently guarding what you put into your mouth. Most Forensic pathologists will tell you that one can profile an individual by analyzing the effects of the meals eaten and the toxic substances injected in the name of food on internal organs and vessels of the diseased. In several cases, we see doctors missing the primary diagnosis of their patients because their pathology is shrouded by the diverse complications brought about by their patient's increase in BMI, cholesterol, etc. Health they say is wealth and as someone striving to be the best at what they do, you should be in tiptop shape at all times and the only way to achieve this feat is to be constantly in good health, earnestly guarding what you eat and drink, watching what you do and treading on the path of caution in your daily living.

"The secret of health for both mind and body is not to mourn for the past, worry about the future, or anticipate troubles but to live in the present moment wisely and earnestly"
Buddha

IV)   YOU NEED ADEQUATE FINANCES

All through my years as a medical student I heard many stories and came across quite a number of individuals that could not complete medical school or dropped out not because they did not have the brains or discipline to study medicine rather because they just did not have adequate finances to do so.

Although personally, I do not think that this factor should be a limiting one, I, however, consider it to be very important. If you don't have strong financial backings or at least a modest one to fit your bills while in medical school, there is no doubt that you will be plagued psychologically, emotionally and spiritually. Needless to say that you are bound to be distracted especially when the stipulated deadline for payments arrives, also you may even find it difficult to afford the relevant textbooks and materials required for a particular course, subsequently, this may influence your grade and hamper you from acing your tests or examinations.

Be that as it may, being financially crippled means you need to work twice as hard. For some odd reasons, it is difficult for those in the medical world to readily get scholarships. They just don't give out things to us on a platter. It is either you get a loan or get a job and work pretty hard.

Of course, there are some medical schools that one may consider as being somewhat affordable. Then again, their affordability, even though relative is seldom skewed by the fact that their standards continue to plummet. Like I said early on, ninety percent of what you learn from medical school, are things that you teach yourself, so what matters is not the medical school that you attend but what you make of the school! In other words, what sort of medical student you become!

 It is no wonder then why some textbooks are considered to be standard regardless of where one is studying. For example, many medical schools around the world use Gray's Anatomy; Keith Moore's Clinically Oriented Anatomy and Last's Anatomy as standard Anatomy textbooks regardless of the university and country Anatomy is being taught. Arguably, this tends to portray a pseudo fixed centralization of information. The major difference and the source of the pseudo believe are the way the information is presented, especially to the novice medical student. This invariably affects the outcome of the learning process albeit be it in a minute way.

Interestingly, one way to bridge this gap is with adequate finances. You may not have money to go study in America but you may be wealthy enough to obtain study materials and books used by your American counterparts. Thus giving you an idea of what is written in American textbooks and knowing their areas of emphasis.

Having a good place to live, a comfortable and conducive place to study is an important pre-requisite for any medical student. Regular meals and adequate means of transportation to and from lectures are luxuries that you can't do without if you intend to succeed as these necessities go a long way in determining not only how your medical journey would look but also its outcome in shaping the type of doctor you eventually become.

My advice to you if you do not have enough money but you stoically desire to be a good doctor is **WORK HARD**. There is no substitute for hard work. If we take a cursory look back through history we see countless stories of people that managed to achieve greatness through hard work even though the odds were stacked against them and they were considered to be of meager means. There is nothing you can't do if you **work hard**.

I often tell my junior colleagues and students, that talents would take you places where finances can't! Someone that is talented and hardworking would nearly always end up in the same place as someone that is financially buoyant, if not better! Granted in some circumstances your finances would take you a distance but your talents would definitely take you all the way, opening doors for you, making you meet and indeed associate with very important people and placing you in a respectable standing among your contemporaries.

In synopsis, to ease the psychological hassle and unnecessary difficulties associated with lack of adequate funds, I suggest if and when possible, ensure you make funds readily available to you before you start medical school.

V)   STRONG FAMILY SUPPORT

Someone once told me that "doctors' kids are more likely to make good doctors themselves". Well, I do not intend addressing the philosophy of this argument but one point we can all agree on is that one of the reasons why kids of medical doctors seem to do very well in medical school is because of the strong support they get from their family and the constant guidance they are shown as they meander through the treacherous paths in the journey of becoming a medical doctor.

My intention here is certainly not to scare anyone without a medical doctor parent, far be it! My own parents are not medical doctors. Rather I only want to underscore the importance of solid family support in one's quest for a medical degree. So do not be afraid. Besides, you have this book and I am convinced that you would do just fine if you adhere to the principles and tenants stated therein. And one of which is that you need a strong family support to succeed in your journey, in other words, you will need someone you can draw strength from within your family niche, by this I mean, someone to urge you on when you are low in spirit or perhaps gravely dispirited, frustrated or challenged by a particular course, lecturer or colleague. For this, there is no substitute for your loving family. Also, you can count on your family to join you in rejoicing when you get that "A" in neurosurgery or maybe curse out that pathology teacher that seems to be giving you a hard time by making it compulsory for you to remember correctly the patho-morphologic concept for every known disease. Whether they understand half of what you say or not, your family can serve as the proverbial "listening ear" to hear you as you lament on the tales that you encounter on your journey.

In so many ways I used this point to my advantage while I was in medical school. You definitely can't imagine how many times I called my folks to tell them about my grades and experiences in medical school. You see, I believed hearing about my exploits made them happy and I constantly wanted them to be happy. So it meant I had to study very hard so that whenever we talked, I had some positive news to tell them. I somehow managed to turn this requirement into motivation for me and I should add that it worked out to my advantage in the end.

I believe that one person that exemplifies the fact that family support plays a tremendous role in influencing the medical journey is Doctor Benjamin Carson, the renowned pediatric neurosurgeon had a mother who constantly positively helped him re-enforced his belief in himself and his ability. By continuously telling him that he could do what others did only that he could do it better, he ended up having great confidence in himself and went on to do and is still doing tremendous things in the field of pediatric neurosurgery. You will be amazed how little words of encouragement can spur one to greatness and the ardent quest to make the world a better place.

The bottom line here is that you should get someone you can share your joys and sorrows with, someone that can remind you of your past victories and encourage you into achieving greater triumphs, because only then will you come to realize what you are truly worth and know that you are not to be judged by your temporary trials, downfall or setbacks.

VI) HAVE A MISSION STATEMENT

As already discussed in the previous chapter it is expedient that as you embark on this journey, you have a solid mission statement. This can be considered as the "what" of your medical journey. Please, take it from me when I say that you don't want to start this journey without having one. In my opinion, it is a grievous mistake, one that I see a lot of medical students make again and again.

You need to know where you are headed and a written statement of that fact cannot be overemphasized. Get a mission statement, memorize it if you may and learn to draw inner strengths from it, certainly, you cannot do without it.

In order not to sound repetitious, I am going to have to refer you to the previous chapter to read about the importance of having a mission statement. Just remember that to get the most from this book you should have a personalized mission statement and chapter two not only tells you how to write one but it illustrates what to do with your mission statement so that it may become beneficial to you. So if you have not gotten one, I suggest you go back to the previous chapter and read it and write one immediately.

"Integrity simply means a willingness not to violate ones identity"

Psychologist Erich F

"I think somehow we learn who we really are and then live with that decision" Eleanor Roosevelt

VII)   HAVE AN ACTION PLAN

This is different from a mission statement in the sense that it is a more detailed description of how you intend achieving discrete parts and indeed all that you have in your mission statement. In other words, if your mission statement refers to the "what" of your journey, the action plan refers to your "how."

A complete action plan would range from daily activities and assignments you set for yourself to the monthly and perhaps yearly compulsory checks to evaluate your progress and see if truly you are on course to meeting the demands of your mission statement.

It is important to know that your action plan should stem from what you hope to achieve with your mission statement, and as such, they should both be in harmony. For example, if you want to be a medical research scientist, in addition to your regular daily studies and class requirement, you should indulge yourself in materials related to medical sciences, and read articles explaining current medical methods of diagnosis and treatment; you should endeavor to know about current breakthrough techniques that make patient care more effective, fast and easier. Also, I reckon you should busy yourself with laboratory findings from all around the world and try to make connections with what you are taught and what you want to achieve and how what your are currently learning can make you a better scientist.

Having an action plan requires discipline. As it mainly relates to doing things on a regular and perhaps daily basis, things that you should never compromise. These are activities that you strongly consider to be the unique source of your happiness, without which your day would remain unfulfilled.

On a personal note, I should tell you that I love books so much, in fact always had from an early age. I am fascinated by the wealth of information hidden within the pages of well-written books. I often liken the feeling to be like going on a treasure hunt, exciting, captivation and blissful especially when you finally get the treasure you seek. In this case knowledge, no feeling in the world can ever beat that!

I cultivated the habit of reading books to the point that if I had not read and learnt something new in a day I would not be happy. You cannot possibly imagine the number of times I got off my bed to go pick up a book so I can get my one new information for the day before I can retire to bed. It was an attitude I cultivated until it finally became a principle for me. Of course, this helped me during my years as a medical student, as I always wanted to learn new concepts and theories daily.

So creating an action plan that entailed daily reading was not much of a problem for me. Nevertheless, I want you to know that you can do the same. Remember to start small and start with things you enjoy doing, or perhaps a course you find particularly interesting. Make it a point to read something about it before you go to bed. And before you know it your habit will soon begin to yield positive results.

The best action plans are those that not only state in detail what you are to do on a daily basis, but they should also stipulate yardsticks to evaluate your progress and determine whether you should get a personal reward or maybe change your course of action.

Just like the mission statement, I believe the action plan is something everyone can and should invest in. With a good action plan, in harmony with your mission statement taking into consideration your school timetable, you can create a structured life that would ensure you have more than adequate time for both academic and extracurricular activities. I can confidently tell you that with an action plan you will discover that your assignments and term papers would be handed in on time and you will be prepared for practically every tests or examination. Most importantly, each day you will see that you are taking baby steps to achieving the set goals in your mission statement.

The most intriguing thing about the action plan is that it is more flexible than the mission statement. You can and should change it from time to time especially when it does not seem to yield the desired effect.

At the start of every semester, equipped with my new timetable in hand, I often draw up an action plan for myself. Stating what I am required to do daily and subjects I am to study with chores and errands that need to be done before the end of the day. As a principle, I try not to make them pile on one another because when they do I feel so overwhelmed and depressed. Weekly, however, I try to evaluate myself, especially with my work, to find out areas of strengths and weaknesses.

Frankly, what I am advocating is something that works. Something that I have tried myself and I have encouraged others to try and interestingly, they have all come back to tell me of the improvement they experienced. You need to learn to take charge of how you spend your day or else, you will have people dump all sorts of frivolities on you. And if you lack structure, you will be forced to join them thereby wasting your time. On the contrary, if you know that there are certain pertinent things that you need to do before you can start that leisure then you will be determined to do all in your power to resist the temptation and do what you have to do when you need to do it. And when you have achieved your goals for the day, if you do decide to go for the leisure spree, you may do it with all you might, having fun even more than the other person knowing that you are in the clear because you do not have any task left un- catered for.

I know that most people have mastered this art. They learn to study well and play, even better. But I want you to understand that in medical school, students are often deceived by these few with the mastery. You never see them study but they are almost always ready for every test and examination regardless of the time. These folks know how to manage their time expertly, they are not the geniuses that we make them out to be, no they just know what to do and how to do it well. So when the time comes to play, they make the most noise and party to the fullest thereby creating the false illusion that this is what they do all day long.

The good news is that you can also be such a person. With a little bit of structure and discipline, I assure you that in no time people will not only marvel at how much you know but will also be in awe at the short time it took you to accomplish much. This is the power of the action plan and daily scheduling.

"A life without purpose is a languid, drifting thing; Every day we ought to review our purpose, saying to ourselves: This day let me make a sound beginning, for what we have hitherto done is naught!"
Thomas A. Kempis

I believe you now know the importance of having an action plan and how it can be beneficial to you perhaps turning you into a genius straight "A" student. So before we go any further I would want you to draw up your own personalized action plan.

To do

i)   Get a plain sheet of paper and a pen
ii) Ensure you have your mission statement, class time table or any other document that will guide your activity throughout this semester.
iii) With the above mentioned documents draw up a personalized time table taking into cognizance the different days of the week, the time you should spend on your different classes, lectures, practices and the discrete goals of your mission statement.
iv) For each day in addition to making provisions for preparing for your subsequent classes you should inculcate activities that would move you closer to your mission statement.
v)   Remember to make room for relaxation. This should be factored in as you draw up your daily action plan and should be considered as a means of reward for something you may have done really well.
vi) After creating the composite time table, take a fresh sheet of paper and write out in form of prose what you are to do daily to achieve your set daily goals. For example you could say:

Continuation

Every Monday;
I will review my notes on embryology and prepare for molecular genetics class. I will also read online the British medical journal on modern laboratory techniques.
As you may have noticed, this states in affirmation all that should be done on Monday and until they are achieved you should deprive yourself of all frivolities and time consuming leisure events.

a) Just like your mission statement, you are to make several copies of your action plan and time table, place them in places that you can easily reach. Also you are to tell your friends and family about them so that they can be supportive as you strive to achieve your goals.

b) Use the action plan as a means to determine where you stand at making your dreams and aspiration come true. By constantly re evaluating yourself. You should ask yourself questions about what you should have done or achieved at the end of each day. This activity you may do on your bed before you sleep, but you must be disciplined and when you discover that there is something lagging or untouched, you are to stand up and do it immediately before going back to bed. If not it may spill into what you are expected to do the next day. This in turn can lead to unnecessary stress and could have been easily avoided.

VIII) HAVE A MENTOR

A mentor can be considered as a wise and trusted counselor. Someone with vast experience in what you intend doing. Therefore, as you start your medical degree journey, it is very important for you to have one. That reliable person you can turn to when you have those numerous nagging questions and confusions that often arise as you embark on this journey.

However, you should know that the type of mentor you have would ultimately determine both what you can get from him/her and how his/her advice affects you. So, it is good to settle for someone easily reachable and almost at your beck and call, someone you can contact anytime to make inquiries as the need arises with the confidence that they would not be offended.

Personally, I suggest that before you make someone your mentor, you should get to know them well enough. Determine their likes and dislikes, noting what things excites them, and those things that they detest would go a long way to curb the unnecessary hurdles you will need to cross as you both make the effort to trust one another.

It is my opinion that you let them know of your willingness to learn from them and how keen you are at being an ardent student. In many ways, it is advantageous to pick a mentor that is a member of the academic staff of your university or college, since, just the mention of your mentor's name or the fact that you associate with him might invoke respect for you too. A point of caution here is that people may equally expect more from you, and as result require you to constantly prove yourself to them.

Be that as it may, you should pick as your mentor, someone you are willing to mirror their life's work and journey. In other words, it is highly beneficial to have a mentor in the particular specialty that you intend joining or one that you have a characteristic flare for. After all, you and your chosen mentor would most likely talk about things that you both have a common interest in. So to ensure that you are in line with what you mapped out for yourself and that your mission statement is upheld I enjoin you to settle for a mentor that can truly answer those pertinent questions about the intricacies on the path you intend treading.

Without an iota of doubt, I strongly recommend that you do let your mentor know about your goals, aspirations and mission statement. As a matter of fact, I advise you to send a copy to them after you have drafted it. Being experienced, they can always provide you with valuable suggestions on how you may go about obtaining your degree without much hassle, by pointing you in the right direction and ensuring you take the shortest route possible.

Of course, I must admit that in certain situations you may find it very difficult to get a suitable mentor in your immediate vicinity, perhaps due to the fact that such relationships are not encouraged, frowned upon, or for some other cogent reasons. If and when this occurs, you may choose a mentor that is not close by or perhaps one that you do not intimately know. Nevertheless, I want you to recognize that you need to get materials from them in the form of books, autobiographies, articles etc. Here again, the idea is simple, all you should do is churn through their materials in search of answers to the challenges that might come your way. The chances are that you are most probably going to find answers to your questions as you go through their works.

I had a friend in medical school that was so fascinated by Doctor Benjamin Carson. He managed to read every printed material by this seasoned physician from "gifted hands" to "think big"....he happened to be so fond of Dr Carson's work that he earned the nickname, "gifted hands". In all honesty, it is that simple! However, although my friend never had the opportunity of personally meeting Dr. Carson his devotion and a strong sense of followership made him capable of mirroring his life to be similar to that of the seasoned physician and therefore, spurring him into venturing to be greater than himself and daring to walk in the footsteps of Dr. Carson. In the end, though, I am convinced that even though my friend may not attain the fame and status of the good Doctor, he definitely would not be far off from the mark.

Also, there is no hard rule that says your mentor should only be a teacher or professor. It could be a senior colleague or student. I discovered that advice from senior colleagues can be very helpful while you are in medical school, especially if you find yourself in one of those schools where teachers don't personally know each student. From your senior colleague, you can learn a lot about a teacher, the way he'll model his classes, tests, and examinations. And also what he expects from students. The caution here is that when you want to make a student or senior colleague a mentor, do pick one that is hard working! If not you may end up having someone that would give miss-guided advice and leave you worse off. Personally, what I did while I was in medical school was to look for a student I knew had an "A" for a particular course and make him/her my informant! I would often bombard him/her with questions about the course, the lecturer, how to best study for classes, what to do right and finally what was his/her take on the subject. I did this so that I could maximize my own learning experience and not make the same mistakes he/she may have made.

IX)   Have Good Books

Frankly speaking, not having good books is synonymous with going to the farm with the wrong implements. Even if you do manage to get the job done, it would be twice as difficult and would certainly take even longer time than expected, not to mention, leaving you with lots of cuts and bruises.

You cannot afford to go through medical school without reading the right books or literature. Given the vast amount of information one is required to grasp in the shortest possible time, and the alarmingly fast manner in which this information changes, coupled with the dilemma of constantly being up to date on current trends and practices in medicine, there is the need to read just the right books.

Certainly, we can all agree that there are tons of medical literature out there, all claiming to be both sacrosanct and comprehensive for medical students in their various fields. The big question then is which ones do you chose?

The answer to this question is simple; before you finally decide what books to buy you should first discover what sort of learner/reader you are. For example, if you happen to be a visual learner you would need to get books with lots of colorful pictures, charts, illustrations, graphs and diagrams. On the other hand, you may be someone that dislikes pictures or diagrams in a text because you believe that they hamper the flow of the material. Then you should go for books with fewer pictures graphs charts etc. what I am trying to say here is that to avoid the unnecessary confusion that is evident when trying to buy a book, several factors must be taken into consideration and one of which is determination of the type of learner you are, because if you do this, you will ultimately obtain maximum use of your study sessions.

Also, you may require more than one book to study. I often tell people that I have a defect, which is, I can hardly ever do a constructive and adequate study with one textbook. I use at least two books for whatever I am studying if I intend to be thorough and effective. As such, I get the privileged to quickly see the discrepancies in the author's viewpoints and notice the different areas of the subject matter where the emphasis is made. Most importantly I often discovered that the chances of the second author answering the questions I have after reading the first material are higher.

Again, I am often asked by students what books are better or best for a particular subject or course. And they are usually bewildered when I tell them, "none". Yeah! It may sound outrageous but it is the truth. The books you should settle for should be based on recommendations from your teachers. After all, you would be eventually graded by them! I advise students to go to their tutors at the start of each session or semester and make enquiries about the textbooks suitable for the course, then haven procured this textbook, they may desire to get a subsequent book that mirrors their learning pattern. You see, from experience, I discovered that students are more prone to ultimately use the second book they got, for the obvious reason that they consider it to be simple, and easy to understand. You may think that I am inconsiderate in asking you to get the second book. But I want you to know that I am not. You should understand that a bulk of what you learn In medical school are things that you teach yourself from books and other sources and if you don't like the textbook you are studying from or cannot totally comprehend what is written therein, how then can you maximize your learning.

There are two types of learning I want you to be aware of, the first being, learning to know and the second, learning to pass examinations. In many ways you will need to study the textbook you are given by your teacher so you can pass your examination and maybe get the excellent "A" grade that you so dearly desire, but if you truly want to know something or perhaps commit it permanently to your memory, you should be learning to know. So that even after your examination, you are still able to reproduce the information and use it as you continue your education.

 I believe every good medical student should carry the mindset of learning to know. I know it may be difficult, plus it requires hard work, eventually, though, I am certain the benefits far outweighs the initial stress. For example, students that practice the learning to know scheme often don't require too much time to prepare for an examination and they always do better when given impromptu tests. Metaphorically speaking, it is pretty much like being ready all the time. So just for the sake of emphasis, I want to say this again, since you will be doing bulk of the studying and indeed learning yourself, I admonish you to get a book that you will be most comfortable with and endeavor to study to know and not merely memorizing data because you want to pass examinations.

Another important point I wish to raise here is that in considering books to buy, you should endeavor to buy books that are globally recognized. These books, I believe have a "leveling effects." In other words, irrespective of where you find yourself and the name of your medical school, you can be confident that you are getting the same information as your contemporaries all over the world. So your location does not seem to matter as you are privy to up to date information about modern trends in medical practices from renowned physicians and researchers. You should only buy books that have become household names in their respective fields. Not to sound like someone making an advertisement, I have decided to make a laconic list of books with global acclamation. Just to give you an idea of what I am talking about.

For example:

Grays anatomy for anatomy

Guyton and Hall for physiology

Robbins pathology for pathology

Harrisons for internal medicine

I am sure thirty to fifty percent of physicians at one point or another would have used one of the above-mentioned texts.

Just before I conclude this segment, I briefly want to talk about the importance of having a comprehensive medical dictionary. One of the things I got when I first got admission into medical school was a medical dictionary. You see, learning medicine is like learning a new language and you can only truly excel as a medical student if you know the true meaning of most medical terminologies and can apply them in patients care. Learning medical vocabulary is an asset. What better place to find more than ninety percent of all words you will ever encounter in medicine than in a medical dictionary? As a matter of fact, my advice is that you always have a medical dictionary with you as you study, this is particularly helpful to person's that are freshly admitted to medical schools and only just started learning medicine with the brazen reality that the words or terminologies are either too strange or somewhat too difficult to fully understand. Equipped with a good medical dictionary and relentless efforts, you will soon begin to, not only understand but quickly get a hang of what you formerly thought was difficult and marveled in awe! One of the reasons I decided to write this book is to demystify medicine and make it clear so that medical students can have a better view on how to navigate through the challenges that enshroud studying medicine, and I believe that the most valuable advice that I can give is that you love your medical dictionary, have it in all forms If necessary; prints, digital, because certainly, you can't do without it.

Finally, I know that some students find it better reading from books written in series, either because of their simple and easy presentation of complex data or maybe it just simply suits the way they learn. If you are such a student I recommend that in addition to the constant use of your particular choice of series, you should get a proper textbook for reference, perhaps one recommended by your professor will suffice here. Since these books written in series may lack the adequate information required for the course or the point of emphasis may be different from your professors.

X) HAVE GOOD AND RELIABLE FRIENDS

Just like embarking on any other journey, the presence of a good friend on the trip to obtaining a medical degree is highly valuable. Of course, you have your classmates and colleagues with you, but it gets to a point where their associations would not be enough and you will long for something more which can only be found in a good friend.

As you may have noticed the caption for this segment is the need to have a good and reliable friend. And if you are wondering why I used both good and reliable in the same statement to characterize the sort of friend you will need, let me tell you, it is for emphasis.

Medicine as a course has a way of taking its tremendous negative toll on any relationship. But it would take a good and indeed reliable friend to understand and certainly accommodate you as you spend your scarce time battling the numerous monsters that lie ahead in your journey to obtain a medical degree. For instance, you may need to go for days or even weeks without contacting your friends, because of your workload and you would need their understanding to keep the flames of your relationship burning by calling, texting, emailing tweeting etc. although you are not able to immediately reply their texts and emails, the simple thought that someone cares for you to the point that they send you these small greetings can turn out to be very soothing.

I should out rightly tell you that your relationships would be far from being symbiotic since you will require more from them than you will be able to give. Hence, to avoid the squabbles that may ensue, you are expected to inform them earlier so that they are not taken aback by your actions.

"Anyone can sympathize with the sufferings of a friend, but it requires a very fine nature to sympathize with a friend's success"
Oscar Wilde

Interestingly, I know for a fact that sometimes friends can serve the same purpose as a family. They can be the spring of emotional support when you are down or depressed, you can call them to cry, complain, scream, wail or do whatever makes you feel better. In like manner, when you experience those moments that you just wish to share with someone special, you can always do so with your friends. Believe me, there would be times when you have some good news to share, but you are not able to share them with your colleagues or classmates. A classic example is if you managed to pass a course and for some reason, others in your class just didn't do so well. You realize that although you are itching to jump and celebrate in joy for your success, you cannot. You are forced to bottle up your emotions as you may be viewed as acting inappropriately. Then you can always turn to your friend and have your chance to not only talk about your triumph but also bask in your glory.

In making the choice of a friend you may want to pick one that is very understanding, and not only know the importance of your dreams but respects and fully supports it. You should settle for a friend that you can reach at any time of the day or night! Someone that would not be offended when you leech on them, because you certainly would! I advise that you make it known to your friends that you will call on them from time to time for support, encouragement and most importantly reassurance.

One mistake I see medical students making is associating with individuals that ultimately derail them from their path. If you must have a companion on this journey, please let it be one that you can trust to put you on track. One that would not have you make decisions that you will end up regretting.

I believe that at the start of any relationships you must set the basis on which the union should flourish. For instance, you could have different buddies for different activities, such as play buddy, study buddy, exercise buddy, music buddy etc, the point here is to strike a balance and ensure that you and your buddies clearly understand the basis of the relationship. Definitely, you cannot eat your cake and have it, there is no point being with the exercise buddy when you should be studying for a test. It is agreeably a recipe for disaster. Seriously speaking, you should learn to properly manage your friends; this includes both friends you have within the academic sphere and others outside.

Among your friends within the medical or academic world, you should be weary of those that directly or indirectly seek to discourage you from studying. Your primary purpose of being in medical school is to study to become a medical doctor any other thing that you may be doing contrary to this is secondary and should not take priority over your studies. There are some that want you to act otherwise! I have already talked a little about these ones, who although have already studied would want to lure you away from your books to go partying or playing with them. As an astute student you should be willing and ready to say NO to the thought of abandoning your books.

Also, there are some who are only interested in acting super cool. These ones are not in any way interested in getting the medical knowledge. As such you often find them complaining about every teacher and May even make you believe that all professors, lecturers, teachers, nurses, and indeed the world, are on a witch hunt to get them. My advice for you is simple. You must flee from them! It is depressing enough to have material of over a hundred pages to churn through in a limited time span, but to have someone nag and bore you throughout is even more depressing and troubling.

It seems logical to have a friend that is optimistic regardless of what obstacles lay ahead. There is nothing like having someone to encourage you and make you strive for greater things in life. No doubt, the amount of strength you can draw from such individual can be phenomenal. In as much as you are ready to accept that there are challenges on this journey, I think you should be excited to know that there is hope for you. So many have embarked on this journey with successful outcomes, definitely your story would not be different. You should listen to everyone but I vehemently advise that you don't take all you hear without logically determining their outcome. Don't get overly bothered by the worries of your colleagues, especially when it is evident that things may turn out differently for you.

"A pessimists sees the difficulty in every opportunity, an optimist sees the opportunity in every difficulty"

Winston Churchill

You may run into students that erroneously feel that they know more than their lecturers. They may go as far as making you feel that the lecturers are always wrong. Granted they can get some information from a textbook, the internet or some reliable source that seems to be different from what the teacher says, but that's no opportunity to be rude or assume your teacher is totally useless. If you associate with such individuals, you stand the risk of being blacklisted. So be careful, you should rather associate with respectable, jovial and loving individuals because your association can ultimately determine people's opinion and attitudes towards you.

The bottom line is that in the immediate vicinity of your medical school, you will need friends that encourage you to be constantly better than you currently are. Especially when they are well aware of the challenges you are facing, you expect them to treat you with more compassion! Personally, I advise that in your immediate environment you should have friends that are students in a class or two ahead of you because you stand a better chance learning from their experiences. They can provide quality recommendations on courses, lectures, lectures etc. all you should do is search for someone that shares similar aspirations as you do, make them your friend and ask them all the questions in the world, from how to best study for individual courses to best study materials at your disposal. Importantly, with their associations you can be shielded from making the same mistakes that they made thus making your sojourn less dramatic. Let me let you in on a little secret, I often got past study questions from my senior colleagues even before the start of the semester, this made my work much easier, because I could study during the holidays and by the time school officially started, I had covered much ground and of course, most of my colleagues and classmates were left in awe! I reckon you should do the same, believe me, it is beneficial. When most of your classmates are perhaps only learning the course or information for the first time, for you, it would be a revision, you would have understood the complex areas of the subject matter and created solid re-enforcement that makes it easier for you to eventually excel in any test or examination. So the key is not just to start on time, but to do so with the most relevant materials, all of which you may procure from your senior colleague or friend.

With respect to friends that you may have outside of the school environment, you should ensure that they are both accommodating and encouraging. Flee from individuals that would rather belittle what you are doing, those that think that your profession is just a waste of valuable time and is perhaps less lucrative! You also should be weary around the so called friends that try to make unfair comparisons with the study of medicine and the study of some less stressful course. Yes, unfortunately, you will have them, people that would wonder why you spend so much time studying and make you feel that the sacrifice is not worth it and you are practically wasting your time. They will tell you that their course is also difficult but they find time for play too. Don't be deceived, medicine is not an easy course to do; you require discipline, determination, encouragement and much more of all that is written in this chapter. If your friends can not support you and make you study well and hard, my advice is loose them! You are in a tasking profession, and as such you need not be surrounded by those that look to compound your burden.

On the contrary, I believe you should be the one influencing them, telling them about the importance of hard work and discipline. For all intents and purposes, let your friends know about your dreams and aspirations, tell them about the lines that you would not have them cross, the most important being relegating your academics. If they are truly your friend, they will be understanding and totally respect your wishes.

It may sound selfish, but I have friends for practically different reasons and activities. For study time, for play, for exercising, for talking politics, for religion, you name it! And my number one rule is to never let them mix. I try as much as possible to compartmentalize my life because I discovered that it was the only way to keep up with my hectic schedule and not complicate matters for myself. And it was relatively easy to turn one person down for another as my need arises, without having to make lengthy excuses or explanations. By doing this, I also discovered that whenever the friend finished serving their purpose, our association dies a natural death. Without any reasonable doubt, I am confident that to a large extent I am in control of my life as I don't have someone overly bugging me with the frivolous activities that can distract the medical student.

Finally, I want to remind you that you should not compromise having friends that understand, support and encourage you. It is almost certain that you may not be emotionally able to give them much, and you will be more dependent on them than they on you. Let them know this, and be ready to severe relationship with those that make you compromise your studies. At the end of the long hard day, the only thing you have at your disposal is the knowledge you manage to amerce while you were in medical school and for this, you will be given a certificate, not for your friendships, or associations, or the parties, or clubs you attended. Make the most of medical school, it is only a limited number of years you need to persevere, don't compromise that which is most important. You are in school to study and not make friends, and study you should, if however, you must make friends, ensure they are good and reliable.

"Dream lofty dreams, and as you dream, so you shall become. Your vision is the promise of what you shall one day be; your ideal is the prophecy of what you shall at last unveil"
James Allen

XI) BE DISCIPLINED
Discipline is one character I suppose every medical student and indeed, doctors, should and must have. Daily as a medical professional, you are saddled with the responsibility to care for human life and you definitely need more than your knowledge in medicine

to undertake this task. You need discipline to practice the precepts and tenants of medicine in a responsible way so that you can be called a successful and explicit physician.

Some individuals have correctly metaphorically described medical study and medical student's life as being in the army. With the overbearing number of rules, protocols, guidance, and regulation for treating and managing the sick, the physician cannot afford to make costly mistakes or engage in unnecessary compromises as this may lead to the loss of life.

As an astute student, you should be willing to forsake all other events or persons for the practice of medicine. Interestingly, society expects this from you since anything short of total commitment is grossly unacceptable. You cannot say you fully grasp and understand the task ahead of you and the willingness to meet its challenges without possessing an ounce of discipline.

One of the advantages of being disciplined is that it gives you the impetus to stay true to your values, dreams, aspirations, and mission statement and action plan. You cannot claim to be disciplined and in anyway relegate your studies or academic for frivolous activities that would be in no way beneficial to achieving your goals or mission statements. It takes discipline to put off going on that date with the beautiful girl that you spent all semester wooing- but instead, settle for preparing for the test you have in a couple of days. Even though the test isn't quite as imminent, you would rather stay back to properly prepare than jump on the opportunity, knowing that when you ace the test you may consider going on the date as your reward. By doing this no matter how badly the date turns out to be, you will have something smile about, your "A"!

A disciplined person knows not to waste his/her time, not to mention, wasting other people's time. It is a well-acknowledged fact that in medical school, time is not just enough. For some odd reason, time is something nearly every medical student and perhaps doctors seem to lack. They often find themselves complaining about no time to do this or that assignment, no time to write and turn in that term paper, no time to prepare for tests and examination, no time to attend lectures, no time to go for practical classes, and no time to be present in ward rounds. So time is overwhelmingly lacked and in dire need. Therefore, I enjoin you to use your discipline to adhere to the limited time you have at your disposal. Indeed, it may sound as a cliché if I say there is time for everything. But in medicine, this maxim cannot be any more buttressed. Take it from me when I tell you that if you do not have an ordered life as a medical student, you will find yourself going through classes and writing exams without properly digesting what you are taught. And before you know, you will be in final year and lack adequate knowledge to show for all your troubles. Undoubtedly, you will end up being scared of not only writing your professional examinations but the thought of practicing may be daunting. Time waits for no one, if you are not adept in doing your assignments and studying what is expected of you, you will sooner than later end up overwhelmed and depressed.

From this discussion, you may have noticed that I mentioned time management as I talked about discipline. This is because it happens to be one area I believe most medical students experience problems. They get carried away doing many things. They know what to do and sometimes, how to do it, but the problem is they lack the discipline needed to not only work with time but be fully determined to follow it to the letter. And not compromise due to some flimsy excuse!

My intention is not for you to see discipline as one intricate concept that resides somewhere in the clouds far from the reach of mere mortals, or as an attitude that is reserved for only the selected few geniuses in our midst. Rather, I want you to see it as something attainable. Everyone can and should be disciplined. Not only does society expect discipline from us all, we are often attracted and charmed by individuals that portray this attribute, even if it is in the slightest of ways, we celebrate them. It's no wonder then that discipline is one of the most important characters a good physician or physician in training should possess.

Most student chuckle when I tell them this, "it takes discipline not to cheat in a test" especially when "others are cheating!" I understand that in medical school it is difficult to succeed without having to bend corners and indulge in activities you would rather never have your patients know. It is even more difficult when this peril is considered to be the norm of the day. You know that although you can't beat them it is unwise to join them. So you do everything in your power to resist the urge or temptations as they come your way and pray to God that you succeed. Seriously speaking in most cases, if you are truly steadfast to your cause and hold firmly your beliefs, no matter how complex the temptations, you will come out on top. Cheating in an examination or test is bad, an obvious fact! It takes someone that is disciplined to overcome this temptation. As I have come to understand, one of the reasons students cheat in examinations is largely because of their fear of failure that stems invariably from lack of discipline. Look, if you are a disciplined person, someone that judiciously follows the schedules and study plans, I am convinced that you will be ready for almost every test or examination you will be given. And the unnecessary fear of failure will be totally uncalled for. It is as simple as that. While a medical student, I often joked that I could never fail any test or examination. I said this emphatically one day that some of my friends thought I was boastful. But it was indeed the truth. I know how much I put into my studies and daily preparations and if I weren't confident I would not make those bold proclamations. Also what they did not understand was that I was not afraid of failing, not because I am a genius and don't make mistake but rather because I have developed a method of dealing with my mistakes or failures, which by the way are few and far between! This secret I am willing to share with you; I believe one of the greatest information hidden from medical students is what to do with mistakes. Rather than spend too much time rejoicing, on what they got right in a test or examination, they should be concerned about what they missed. It is my experience that what is missed, if not properly sorted and understood could one day later come to hunt one. Personally, I make it a point of duty to always go back to my teachers after every examination to not only inquire about my grades but also see the questions I got wrong. I discuss the wrong answers with my teachers and make a note to self never to make the same mistakes again in the future. They say people learn better when they have an emotional link to what they are learning. It is true and you can readily make emotionally links by using my method and going over the questions you failed. Reviewing it if necessary and knowing or understanding the most appropriate response is always beneficial in the long run. It makes you a better student and one less likely to repeat the same mistakes.

Well, you may be thinking that discipline is just one trait you just don't seem to possess. Yes, you love to study, you want to be successful, and you know the importance of what lies ahead because you can see the big picture, but you just cannot seem to bring yourself together to do what needed to be done. If this is you, I want to say, don't worry. There is a way out, the trick is taking all the huge tasks before you and cutting them into tiny bits and pieces that can be easily managed. For instance, you may not have the zeal to study twenty-four seven, but you can just tell yourself you will study every other day, or perhaps consider renaming some days of the week as study days or subject days. And you are not to embark on any other activities until you have accomplished those you set out to do for the day. And when you do accomplish you task, you give yourself a treat. Of course, it is important to space out the treat so that they would be something that you often look forward to with great enthusiasm and as a catalyst to spur you into repeating the task some other time.

We can always tell disciplined medical students when we see one. They are very easy to spot since they are those that hand in their assignments on time; they are always ready for every class, test or examination. They don't cheat in tests, they fully participate in practical lessons and they display adequate knowledge in whatever they are required to know. All these traits you can have if you can only resolve to follow through with your daily plans and schedule, If you determine not to allow anyone, anything, or any activity get you derailed from your desired path, if you are willing and ready to fix your eyes solely on the goals and not be cajoled by the frivolities around. Then, in the end, your price would not only be discipline but the actual realization that you are an esteemed student and physician, what is best, your achievement came by you enjoying what you do!

"Nothing in this world can take the place of persistence. Talent will not; nothing is more common than unsuccessful people with talent.
Genius will not; unrewarded genius is almost a proverb.
Education will not; the world is full of educated derelicts.
Persistence and determination alone are omnipotent.
The slogan "press on" has solved and always will solve the problems of the human race"
Calvin Coolidge

XII) BE TOLERANT

It is often easy to forget that every person is unique, and as such, we all possess certain unique traits and characters. It is, however, therefore obvious that we cannot all learn at the same pace or understand complex principles at the same level all at once. Some people will grasp information faster than others! So it is very important to be tolerant; you should exhibit tolerance for yourself, for others and for situations, especially those you don't seem to have any control on. Tolerance is, in essence, a trait you will require to succeed as a medical student or doctor.

I have given you some secrets and pointers to help you succeed and indeed, I would still give you more valuable information as you continue to read this book, so that your experiences and struggles in your quest for procuring a medical degree is both befitting and bearable. But in light of our current discussion, you should understand that this empowerment is not a right to scorn those that are not opportune to have the same information as you do. You are not to loathe or lord yourself over them or make them feel inferior in any way. Rather you are advised to be sympathetic to their plight and do everything in your powers to help them, especially when they seek your counsel.

I am certain that by the time you are done reading this book, and while you practice the precepts stated therein, you will, in no time be transformed into the model student with your friends and colleagues dotting all around you in awe and reverence that they would soon begin to come to you for advice. I expect you to be humble and teach them the principles you learnt from this manuscripts. You are learning these secrets not because you want to keep them to yourself, no, I want to kindle a fire inside you that would shine brightly for the world to see. And the best way you can be that bright light that illuminates the paths of people is by teaching them the things you learnt from this book, the very things that shone brightly on your path.

Even as a medical doctor, there is tremendous need to show tolerance as you go along your daily affairs. Tolerance towards your patients, nurses, senior and junior colleagues is a prerequisite. In practice, you will come across many patients that would ask a whole lot of questions concerning their treatment or management. It is your duty to accommodate their questions and be sympathetic to their concerns and alleviate the fears they raise. Whether it is right or wrong! Also, you may have patients that would blatantly refuse to follow the recommendations that you give to them and even lie about steadfastly adhering to them. When you find out, if you are not tolerant, you may lose your temper and patients end up branding you as an uncaring doctor. Invariably on the long run this is most definitely bad for your practice or career.

As already mentioned, you need tolerance to relate with your colleagues or nurses. You should realize that although they may be lower members of the medical staff hierarchy, they play an important role in the overall care for patients. Instead of constantly screaming and abusing them, it is your duty to encourage them and ensure that they become better in all that they set out to do. It is well-known fact that an amiable working environment breeds efficiency from all.

Interestingly it is so easy for doctors to forget that they are only humans, hence, bound to make mistakes. They carry themselves with this gigantic pride that it becomes difficult for them to be tolerant of anyone, including themselves! I am not advocating that doctors think very little of one another or condone their errors, certainly not! Rather what I am saying is that they should be more tolerant of themselves.

It makes no sense to be your own personal slave driver, you should learn to make room for relaxation and recognize that all work and no play would most likely make Jack the dull boy. In your quest for the medical degree, you should be tolerant enough to yourself and seize the opportunity to go for walks, acknowledge nature, smell roses, swim seas, sit in gardens and just, live life!

No matter what is going on around you, in as much as you put in your best, you should be confident that in the end, it will all pan out for good in your favor. So there is really no need to be foolishly anxious. Tolerance is what you need. I knew of a colleague who lost his mind while we were in medical school, and it was rumored that it happened because he drove himself so hard while preparing for an examination. In the end, he couldn't write the examination and was eventually demised from the program. The morale here is to do things in moderation. Have a solid plan in place, and when things don't go the way you expected, be confident that you did your best and re-evaluate your actions, noting the areas you missed or messed up, and then come up with ideas and recommendations for doing things better. By shifting the focus from your failures to how you can better yourself, you will learn to be more tolerant of you.

Just so you don't get too carried away by the journey you are about to embark on, and perhaps forget certain important items, I have taken the pains to draw up a checklist for you. Be sure to go through this list and ensure that you have all that is demanded before you continue on the trip. Since, I would not want you stopping on the way because you left some important item behind.

The things you require for the journey

- A SOUND MIND
- RECORGNISE YOU WILL MAKE MISTAKES
- GOOD HEALTH
- YOU NEED GOOD FINANCES
- YOU NEED STRONG FAMILY SUPPORT
- YOU NEED A MISSION STATEMENT
- YOU NEED AN ACTION PLAN
- YOU NEED A MENTOR
- YOU NEED TO HAVE GOOD BOOKS
- YOU NEED GOOD AND RELIABLE FRIENDS
- YOU NEED TO BE DISCIPLINED
- YOU NEED TO BE TOLERANT

CHAPTER FOUR

THE TYPICAL CHALLENGES OF A MEDICAL STUDENT AND REASONABLE TIPS ON HOW TO FACE THESE CHALLENGES

I bet by now you are already packed for the trip, and I am hoping that you have all that is required to make this voyage a memorable one. So it is time for us to talk about the possible stops, turns, and twists that we are bound to encounter on this journey.

I am excited about this chapter, you should too: because this is where I get to tell you about the hurdles that lie ahead, and give you well-seasoned pointers so that you can easily scale them as they come your way.

Let me start by stating at the onset that different medical schools possess their own unique challenges. In other words, the challenges for a medical student in the

United Kingdom may be different from those that study in South Africa. However, regardless of where you are studying medicine, there are some stresses that are uniform, in the sense that every medical student must experience it irrespective of the part of the globe they are located. One of such stresses is:

The Cumbersome Work Load:
As a medical student, there is no doubt that you will have much to study. There is a whole chunk of data you are expected to go through in four or six years, depending on where you are studying for your medical degree. This is something they often fail to tell you, or perhaps if and when they do, you don't seem to understand the gravity of what they are saying. Before graduation, the average medical student reads close to thirty to fifty textbooks and a whole lot more of handouts, articles or medical journals. So if you are someone that has not already cultivated the habit of reading, I suggest you do so immediately, because from the moment of your matriculation, the countdown begins, you will be expected to voraciously devour information at the speed of light and you can only be truly successful if you have a natural flair for reading.

One of the main reasons studying medicine is even more cumbersome is because there is this constant ebb in the flow of information. On a regular basis, theories are propagated and disproven. And what is worse, society often expects the average medical student to be well aware of the changes that occur in medicine especially since a large majority of them are geared towards patients care and management. To get a clear picture of how fast information, protocols and management schemes changes in medicine, you should be aware of one of a common statement they tell medical students sooner or later during the course of their studies, which is, "some of the things that you read, study or are taught in medical school, would most probably change, be updated, disproved, or abandoned in five or six years time". In other words, protocols, management schemes and recommendations for patient care would be different from what you were taught in your first year by the time you get to your final year. And the most intriguing part of it all is that you are expected to be aware of the changes as they occur. This task, though at first sight may seem Un-do-able. But in reality, it is something you can do, if and only if you can develop the habit of constantly studying.

Another way you can comfortably deal with the cumbersome workload of medical school is to acknowledge that each material you learn often builds on another. You should not see them as discrete entities rather consider them as steps that lead one into another. As a matter of fact, most of your courses would be done in steps or stages anyway! You must transcend from one step to another. But it is important to take each and every step seriously. As it turns out, if by any chance you miss a step or do not adequately understand it before moving to the next step, there is a chance that you will have problems. Since the subsequent steps are usually higher and more difficult. It, therefore, makes complete sense to properly grasp the subject matter of a step before venturing into the other complex parts of this gigantic puzzle. The mistake I find so many medical students make is that they neglect the initial or preliminary part of their studies. Many of them don't start quality studies until their third or fourth year in medical school, by which time they would have missed out on the opportunity of understanding the background or foundation of medicine. Before they know it, they are thrown into doing very complex reasoning and because of their poor background, they find it difficult to comprehend what they are being taught and therefore perform poorly in final test or examination.

This is the reason why it is beneficial to carry the mindset of a fighter from the start of your medical journey, right from matriculation. You should brace yourself for the battles you are to fight, the most important being the enormous amount of information you are required to study. Take it from me, you cannot go through medical school not studying, if you do, you will sooner than later discover how handicap you have become because you will know nothing! Some have dubbed this category of students the liability of the medical world. No doubt, if this persists, depression and frustration would swiftly set in. And you will begin to wonder and ponder how you got yourself in the mess in the first place.

The good news is that I have already given you all that you need to face this challenge. If you read the previous chapter and indeed pack your bag as directed, you will discover that you are equipped to meet this challenge. In any case just as a reminder, to overcome this challenge and be truly victorious, you need: a comprehensive timetable, Discipline, Good and reliable friends to spur you on, and a mentor- just to mention a few. All these you have at your disposal and you may bring out at any moment in time that you are faced with the problem of a cumbersome workload.

Of course from the above-stated arsenal, one factor that cannot be over emphasized is the need for an action plan or a comprehensive timetable or schedule for your daily activities with clear descriptions of what you are to do or achieve before the end of each day. Also, you need a spice of discipline so that you don't make frivolous compromises that further compound the stress of a bulky workload. In like manner, you need a mentor to guide you as you face the different forms the workload challenge may take. Their input should be instrumental in alleviating the stress of medical study, as they can provide you with information that could make you get tasks done in the shortest possible time. Or provide you with the best methods for reading or remembering complex information.

Isolation:

Unfortunately, medicine happens to be one of those courses that steal your social life from you. As a medical student, you discover that you usually don't have ample time to invest in most of your relationships and as such you are often left isolated. Your books can and will keep you from your family, friends and loved ones. In simple terms, you will be deprived of a social life.

You should realize that people often experience this challenge on different levels and it is often very difficult to thread the thin line that exists between studying medicine and not being isolated. In the struggle to overcome the effect of isolation caused by medical school, some individuals end up making compromises on their daily action plan or ultimately altering their mission statement and negatively impacting on their workload.

It is clear that isolation in itself is a trap. Personally, I believe that isolation can be managed and is definitely not too much of a bad thing. Then again, I am often considered a recluse. But to be candid, I think that this is a small price to pay if you want to be totally successful. Besides, sometimes, it is inevitable as you will require isolation to get any valuable reading done. In as much as it would be impossible for you not to encounter isolation, it would be beneficial if you can look for a way to cushion the effect of isolation and make it work in your favor.

Without any doubt, we can agree that it is frightening when we don't find anyone to tell about the events in our lives, the frustrations, the challenges etc. and it is even more disastrous when we lack that shoulder to cry on, when there is none to encourage, console and indeed pull you off out of depression. These are the periods when the perils of isolation take root. The times when you would wish you had a social life. No surprise then, that in desperation, so many medical students make irrational decisions and compromises to curb this problem. Nevertheless, as already stipulated in the previous chapter, to win this battle of isolation as a medical student, you will require both a strong and adequate family support plus the presence of good and reliable friends, because it takes your family and friends to remain sympathetic and understanding when you fail to contact them. And still be supportive, encouraging you if and when you require their help. My personal trick to fighting isolation is having friends for different purposes. That way, you can always easily reach out to any of them anytime you want and one can always take the place of the other.

"When plans are laid in advance, it is surprising how often the circumstances fit in with them"
Sir William Osler

Emotional Distraction:

This is another area where I often see many medical students stumble and fall prey. Especially when they are faced with isolation! In other words, to fight the reality of loneliness and isolation, they get emotionally involved with someone. Not saying that this is entirely bad, but if not properly managed, I consider this a time bomb waiting to explode. Certainly, I say emphatically, that if possible, you should not be emotionally involved with anyone while in medical school. If you can avoid it, then do! Emotional entanglement can take a detrimental toll on you.

You must understand that you have only but a limited time to spend in medical school, although it has the tendency of feeling like a lifetime! But in no time you will be through with medical school and you have your whole life ahead of you with more than enough time to love and be loved in return.

I know that some may argue that it does not really matter how, when, and where you fall in love, and that being emotionally involved with someone while in medical school is not much of a terrible thing! To them, I say more power to your elbows! Nevertheless, even though, I partially agree with this school of thought, I wish to reaffirm that since there are so many uncontrolled variables and uncertainties that characterize being emotionally involved with someone, it is unwise to do so while in medical school. For instance, you can't afford to be in an abusive relationship, with the hope of working things out while you study medicine. Or be in a relationship where your partner does not support or recognize the importance of what you do or the journey you are on. You just can't function in such an environment. In the end, you will accumulate more pressures in addition to those you already have by mere virtue of being a medical student. Imagine going through a breakup while you have to prepare for an important test or examination? Or perhaps that examination is your Boards or professional examination? Believe me, it is not worth it. To avoid the drama and unnecessary charade, please do not get emotionally involved with anyone. If you are destined to be with that girl or guy, you will be. It may take some time, but destiny would eventually take its course. This is one area where I expect you to be calm and humble. Do not be deceived by your age, sex, or status. As long as you have decided to thread this path, you should be willing and ready to adhere to the sacrifices that are expected. And just like we dealt with isolation, you can get platonic friends and foster good relationships that may be generally symbiotic without having the complexities of emotional entanglements.

Social Challenge:

Just like emotional entanglements, medicals students are faced with enormous social challenges. This is evident in the fact that the somewhat busy medical student's schedule makes it practically impossible for them to be social animals. As a matter of fact, it is quite common to see medical students rightly pride themselves as introverts! A unique trait they develop because of their cumbersome workload and nature of the medical program. Between running around for lectures, practices, classes, they don't have the time to go enjoy the numerous pleasures or life, especially when the pressures of medicine come crashing on them. Certainly, you realize sooner or later as a medical student, that to succeed, you should be willing to temporarily let go of these niceties and pleasures. I had a lecturer that often reminded us that if we were to be outstanding in our career and work as physicians, we should be ready to forfeit the pleasures of life and indeed the things that make us social animals while in medical school. According to him, when we left medical school, we had all the time in the world to not only make friends but truly bound with them without the guilt of worrying about undone tests, assignments or examinations.

Sincerely speaking, this challenge is not only obvious, but it is also considered as a rite of passage for every medical student. If you have not gotten to the point where your friends and perhaps family accuse you of neglecting them or not being able to meet an obligation or engagement because of your workload, I am convinced that you are probably not properly doing what is expected of you. Or perhaps it will happen sooner than you expect! It is inevitable, you will turn down engagements from your friends and they will complain.

You may find it frustrating to see your friends from other disciplines attending parties, nightclubs and doing the things that you so long to do. Well, no matter how frustrating or challenging it may be, you are not to succumb to the pressures. Since this is one of the sacrifices you have agreed to make when you chose medicine, or perhaps when medicine chose you! Either way, to fully realize your potential, be certain that aspects of your life would suffer. It is advisable to let your social life be on a temporary halt until you at least get a solid footing in your studies and if you are someone that is easily influenced, I suggest you totally put off having a social life until you have completed your medical study. Believe me, in the long run, it is not an expensive price to pay.

To beat the challenge of social burden or its lack thereof, I devised a pragmatic system. When I have a social function to attend to, I use what I call the alternative variable to critically analyze my options. I weigh the pros and cons of going to a function with those of studying at the same time. And I ask myself, that giving my current emotional and psychological state, if I stayed behind would I achieve much studying? In other words, if it is certain beyond any reasonable doubt that I would not get any fruitful reading done, I just may go for the social gathering- and by the way, I should add that my social engagements were gravely streamlined. I was either attending a friend's birthday, going on a date, or attending special ceremonies organized by the school such as convocations or matriculations. So the limited engagements at my disposal made it quite easy for me to follow my schedule and routines without feeling guilty turning down events that clashed with my short term plans.

It would be impractical for me to end this section about social challenges without mentioning that there are some individuals that have mastered the act of balancing their academic work with their social life. Indeed these few individuals buttress the point that man is a social being and it is unfair and albeit, unwise to totally neglect this aspect of our existence. My rationale is that if you are sure that being a social animal will in no way affect your existence and study of medicine then I may permit that you combine the two. But if however, you discover that you are struggling to put on appearances and thereby constantly compromising your academics, then, I suggest you let go of your social life, especially since it would only be for a limited time. Eventually, when the time is right, you will move with the prestigious crowd that you so long for now.

Like I have said before, your primary purpose of being in medical school is to have a medical degree and become a doctor, and most definitely not because you want to make friends or become a social monkey. If by any chance you have event or events occupying the place of this task, you are advised to forfeit such. This singular act can be the determining factor for making you an outstanding physician. So take it seriously, it may be difficult at first, especially when everyone seems to be doing it, but remember, you are not everyone, you are you! Someone special, with unique hopes and aspirations, daily you strive to meet your expectations, don't let what people think, say or feel deter you from doing what you need to do. Be wise, put the extra effort to be the best you can be and in the end, you will be glad you did. As your discipline will pave way for you as you strive for excellence as both a medical student and practicing physician.

The Cost of Medical School:

This is an obvious challenge, medical education all over the world is considered expensive. You are likely to pay more in terms of tuition if you decide to be a medical student. The irony is that in most cases, the money you pay can be justified, in other words, when you dig deeply you would agree with the fees you are being forced to pay. Then again, one often wonders why there is a discrepancy in the prices if medical education. Where in some places it costs a fortune and in others, it is only a token! The bottom line here is not the cost but the quality of education which in several ways is closely related to the cost. That is to say, the quality of education you get is dependent on the amount you pay as tuition. However, in so many institutions of medical learning, you discover and understand why governments pitch in to help reduce the cost of training physicians.

Interestingly if one is financially incapable of paying their way through medical school, there is the tendency of being plagued by a host of troubles. Most important of which include the detrimental psychological strain that can cripple an individual, hampering their learning and ultimately the process of becoming a good doctor. You will need money to buy good textbooks, purchase the relevant and recommended materials, money to photocopy handouts; lecture materials, past questions or study questions, money to buy equipment such as stethoscope, a sphygmomanometer, thermostats, money for laboratory coats, surgical suits and slippers, money to enroll and pay for programs that would help improve your clinical skills and give you an edge over your contemporaries.

Also, you need money to feed and live comfortably or else you will find it difficult studying. You need cash for transportation especially if your medical faculty is located far from your hostel or accommodation. Basically, you need money for everything!

Given the foregoing, it is no surprise to find medical students in debt right after their degree or students that are advanced in age, who already possess some working experience or currently hold two or three jobs while in medical school- just to pay their bills.

The cost of medical school is as difficult as the medical education. That is why you are encouraged to work extra hard. I know a number of students that use this as a motivation. They know that they can't afford to make mistakes so the buckle up and do their best as medical students. Generally speaking, though, every medical student should work hard and even harder when it is evident that it costs a fortune to be trained as a doctor. You should flee from being mediocre.

I should let you know that most medical students understand the importance of having money while studying medicine since they see and indeed feel it first hand from the start of their medical education. With the need to procure relevant textbooks and study materials ever lurking in their faces, or as already mentioned, the need to attend special/additional training course- which is usually expensive! The funny aspect of it all is that, even when you manage to pay your tuition and bills in medical school before you are registered as a professional or physician, you are still expected to write and indeed pay for your professional examination,

Which by the way, is often very expensive too. Such is the life of a medical student, hence the uttermost need for adequate finances!

It is, of course, obvious that the earlier stated premise of working and saving some money before starting medical school is a good way to go about overcoming this hurdle. This remains true because even though you may easily hold a job while in medical school, it can be a daunting ordeal. However, I know a number of individuals that did manage to balance the stress of studying medicine and earning a living. They are the first to intimate you of the numerous difficulties they face. I have tremendous respect for these ones. No doubt it is a herculean task, certainly possible but not advisable.

Inadequacy of Relevant Medical Literature:
Knowing what to study is one big problem most medical student's face. There is an alarming rate of transformation in medical information, and keeping abreast of these changes is definitely a problem, one which is masked by the creation of numerous medical materials with slight alterations. Certainly, for someone new to the medical scene, it is most confusing and debilitating as you are suddenly overwhelmed by the vast amount of information at your disposal to be grasped. To top this up, you are told that the information is not enough and you are given additional sources! In the end, you become more confused as you learn that ninety percent of what you are taught to be true and or correct would be modified by the time you start your medical practice, nevertheless, you are still required to know them or perhaps have an idea of the previous recommendations in medicine. Phew! You may be saying to you self, "it just never stops", but this problem can be tackled squarely and I have already given you the most realistic way to overcome this dilemma.

You can start by asking your lectures or departments for recommendations of the most relevant textbooks for your courses. Fortunately, you can get this information on the websites of many universities. Having gotten these textbooks, your next task would be to procure reference books on subjects you are currently undertaking. This is important because you would need to be abreast of information that is considered as world standards and also knows what your contemporaries around the globe are studying. In other words, since it is quite easy for different authors to emphasize different areas in a subject, with a good reference you, you should be able to connect the dots and become well informed.

After obtaining a reference book, if you discover that both the books your department or lecturer recommend and the one you picked as a reference don't match up with your study method or personal study technique, I suggest you get a separate book that does! However, in most cases, you would be lucky to find books that satisfy both criteria.

I often encourage students to develop the habit of reading medical articles and journals. As a medical student, I subscribed to quite a number of medical journals. The interesting thing now is that you can have an online subscription where different journals and medical bodies send regular updates on various parts of medical discoveries and developments. What I did was to make them send me updates on topics and courses I was currently facing in school. This helped me because as I answered questions in class, I did not only talk about things I read from my textbook, but also of things that are novel in the medical scientific world and have only just been introduced into that medical arena. To be candid, this impressed many of my professors as they were most often glad to see a student interested in modern developments in their respective fields. What you need to understand is that it would take a couple of years before what I read from these journals or articles found their way into the regular standard books, as most of them are reprinted or edited every two to four years. So it felt good to be way ahead of my books!

Another method I used to gauge the knowledge I obtained in medical school is to constantly ask myself certain questions. I often asked what I actually knew and could remember after a class or a course, what I was supposed to know, what my contemporaries in the world knew? By doing this, I could give an adequate evaluation of myself and if need be proffer a different or most suitable course of action.

Although there are quite a number of literature and books out there, I am afraid to say that a vast majority of them are either too, simplistic and void of relevant information, or in other cases, verbose and filled with errors and materials that are ill-suited for the medical student. Your greatest problem will be striking a balance. You will need a book that contains the relevant information for a medical student, written in you unique study style. In other words, these should be books with lots of pictures or diagrams for the visual learner, and books with a succinct explanation in plane and free flowing words for the auditory learner or creation and use of audio books. I believe that this makes the study of medicine bearable, to have books or series of different texts that meet the needs of almost all types of learners. Anyway, because this is not the case, it is your responsibility to not only determine what works best for you but to also find the relevant textbooks that meet your study needs so that you can get the most appropriate information available.

For all of your days in medical school, the greatest investment you can have is the investment is good books. In fact, make your books your best friend, and make good books your closest pals. You can't possibly imagine how many times I went without food so that I could purchase that particular book that suits my study pattern, especially because my school's policy was to provide books for their students. It was not long before I discovered that I could not solely depend on them as their books seldom satisfied my study pattern. So I had to get my own materials! This was the sacrifice I had to pay, though difficult sometimes, in the end, I am glad I did.

If you noticed I captioned this segment the inadequacy of relevant medical literature. This was deliberately done because although there are medical books, some of which you may have, you will soon discover that they may no longer be standard texts or you won't consider them suitable for your study method, hence, the inadequacy of relevant medical texts.

The problem of Time:

This is perhaps one of the greatest burdens recounted often by medical students. It's no secret that it takes a very long time to obtain the medical degree. On average, you spend about ten to twelve years to become a doctor. Even though the actual process of active medical schooling is from four to six years, you are most often required to obtain a pre-medical degree from a college in a course allied to medicine. This can range from two to four years and after medical school you are expected to join a specialty!

Undoubtedly, its takes a long time, and you should be physically, psychologically and spiritually ready for this long ride. What I tell students when they complain about this is to consider the time spent in getting a degree as an investment, one they make now but wait years to reap the rewards.

 One mistake you can make as a medical student is to compare yourself with students of other disciplines, for instance, medical students comparing themselves with someone in the arts or information technology disciplines. These are fields that require relatively less time and resources to obtain a degree, and for some odd reasons, individuals that embark on these courses start the rat race of life faster than most medical students in the same age category. In my penultimate year in medical school, I noticed that most of the students in other disciplines that were in the first year of college with me had already started working; quite a handful had families: married with kids, while I was still engrossed with studying for my final examination. Of course, sometimes I felt bad and wondered what my life would have been if I had chosen another field and if this journey would ever end. But what I later discovered was that the moment I started working as a doctor, I did not only meet up with them but I can also boast that I overtook quite a number of them.

As medical students chances are that you will also experience this, I want you to know that there is hope so don't be dismayed. It would help to have your mission statement at hand most of the time, so you can look at it and become consoled when the burden of time befalls you.

Comparatively, you should understand that although it may seem like getting the medical degree is a long strenuous process, it would be shocking that you will come to see that time is not enough to do the things you are required to do. Such as meeting up with your daily schedules, studying and memorizing assignments and lecture notes, attending classes and lectures, you will just need more time. Hence I often tell students that it is pertinent to maximize the time spent in medical school so that time would not seem inadequate. They should not be found wanting in the area of time management, since if they are it is a possible that they would end up spending even longer time in medical school in form of repeated semesters or years. I have heard about individuals that spend eight years for the four to six years medical degree, the reason for this is not farfetched, they were not meticulous with their time, and so they failed and had to repeat a particular year several times. I am sure you don't want this to happen to you, that is why I say, get a daily schedule and stick to it! Do your tasks and assignments, study promptly so that you would not need to spend a longer than expected time to obtain your medical degree.

Now you may only be in the first year, but before you know it, you will be in the final year, with the scary thoughts of graduation and patient management lurking around the corner, acting as a constant plague to your subconscious. You can become confident at this point, if and only if you managed your time well as a student.

By now you should know that the most important gift you could give yourself as a medical student is learning to properly manage your time so that your stay in medical school can be both eventful and enjoyable. You don't want to see it as too long or too short but just appropriate. The idea is to like what you do and relish every moment that comes your way. Ensure that you don't fall under the group of individuals that are just floating through medical school but be among those that are living life as a complete and competent medical student, gasping all you are being taught and laying solid foundations that will eventually make you a better doctor in the nearest future.

Poem by Og Mandino, "The Greatest Salesman in the World"

How do I change?
If I feel depressed I will sing.
If I feel sad I will laugh.
If I feel ill I will double my labour.
If I feel fear I will plunge ahead.
If I feel inferior I will wear new garments.
If I feel uncertain I will raise my voice.
If I feel poverty I will think of wealth to come.
If I feel incompetent I will think of past success.
If I feel insignificant I will remember my goals.
Today I will be the master of my emotions.

Difficult school Authorities:

Like every other educational institution where students view their school authorities as being nefarious, the medical school as an educational establishment is no different. There is the possibility that members of the school board would be out rightly wicked or not sympathetic to their student's plights: with students unfortunate to have terrible timetables, with clashing lectures, practices at odd hours, examination dates that make it simply impossible for students to cram the night before and so on.

In medicine, it is expected that you are able to meander through all that is thrown at you. In this journey, you will be tested, your zeal, your strength, your ability to persevere and most importantly write and pass examinations would be put to a test. Yes! You will write many examinations, some you will consider more difficult than others. And only two things will be important, the first one being what score or grade you get from the examination and the second what you manage to learn from the course. In the ideal sense, the grade is supposed to be a reflection of what you learnt from the course. So whether the examination dates are conducive or not, you will still be judged on both fronts, therefore, you should endeavor to be steadfast in your preparations and watch your confidence grow in every situation.

"It is not because things are difficult that we do not dare, it is because we do not dare that they are difficult"
Seneca

I should have you know that although it seems realistic to believe that school authorities are on a witch hunt to get students this is usually not true. On the contrary, they are actually there to help you. You should learn to form a rapport with members of your school authority. I say this because I am confident that you are or will be a model student (after reading this book!) you see, model students are often celebrated. Nearly everyone wants to associate with them- even the so-called "difficult" school authorities! Make yourself known to your dean, and other members of the administrative staff, so that when you are faced with any difficulty they can personally make it a point of duty to help you.

The mindset you should have , of your school officials is that they are nice, and pleasant individuals positioned to be of assistance to you in your time of need, even when they act in ways that seem inconsiderate. You should know that ultimately they have your best interest at heart and it is your duty to discover ways that you can work amicably with them regardless of the situation. Let me be clear here, I am not saying that you condone difficult officials, far be it! Rather I am advocating that you put yourself in the position where you are immune to whatever vice that they may have for students. If you come across lazy officials and develop a relationship with them on a personal level chances are that you will have your way with them most of the time, and if they understand that something is important for you, they would eventually act in ways to favor you.

Finally, you will hear about students that will be expelled or punished because they were not in good terms with the school officials. They fall victim to things that ordinarily would have been overlooked if they were model students or in good stead with their difficult school officials.

"Life is like a piano. What you get out of it depends on how you play it"
Tom Lehrer

Difficult Teachers:

A major challenge that you will inevitably face as a medical student is the presence of highly difficult teachers. I am sorry to tell you that you will come across teachers that would never believe that you can know more than them in a particular area, or others that would not want you better than them, teachers that would be threatened by your talents and abilities. Some will hate you because of how you talk, walk or even sit! And some others would be outright racists or tribalistic!

Please know that I am not saying this to scare you, rather, I want you to be prepared. I want to inform you so that you can easily spot these difficult teachers and know how to deal or relate with them.

You see, I once had a very difficult lecturer, who stood in front of my class and declared that nobody would ever have an "A" in his course because according to him, "A" was for God, "B" is for him and "C" is for the masses. How insane is that you are wondering! Every year he makes the examinations more difficult and reduces the duration required to complete the questions. When I heard his declaration, I took it as a challenge, I told myself that I was going to get an "A" and become his God! Well I didn't get the "A", but no one in my class did, I happen to be one of the four students that managed to get "B". I guess what I am trying to say is that it is inevitable for you not to encounter difficult teachers. You will find them around you taking different forms. They would include those that are unfazed and even happy when more than half of their students fail or barely pass their courses. Certainly, you will hear about these ones and when you do, I want you to act like me. Take up their challenge, do your best and surprise them. You have all it takes to be great, you have and know the secrets of success as a medical student, you have all you need to become an outstanding doctor, you have this medical guide, so don't let anyone make you feel otherwise! When a difficult teacher challenges you, I want you to reach into that backpack, the one I made you pack in the third chapter of this book and come up with something that can make you easily overcome the test that is placed ahead of you. This could be in the form of daily revision of your action plan, a strong family support, support from a mentor, very good books and so on. Do not be afraid, dig deep, into your arsenal and you will be just fine.

Apart from having teachers that are less concerned about how students fare in their courses or examinations, you may encounter a different group that shows bias when it comes to grading the knowledge of their students. They rarely know their student's capabilities as such they end up giving random grades. Ultimately you discover that student that don't study or perhaps have little or no idea about the course end up with better grades than those who are hard working and actually understand what the course is about. The irony in this scenario is that most times you cannot be totally pissed with them because you may still need to get in touch with them for another course or semester and you can't be pissed with your lazy classmates for getting better grades because it is not their fault but the teacher's nonchalance! In any case, I believe the best way to avoid this dilemma is to let your teachers personally know you, preferably on a first name basis. This is especially advantageous in a large sized class, where sometimes teachers don't even have the time to go through all the scripts they are given to mark and grade. If they know you, you may have the chance to prove your worth and make them respect your abilities and drive. So when it's time to award marks, they would not forget your exploits and the impressions you may have made on their minds would be solidly imprinted in their subconscious. Giving them something they get to remember, something positive that would eventually work in your favor.

Also for some reasons, you may find it difficult to attend some lectures and classes, if your university is one where attendance of lectures and practical classes are sacrosanct as they take up a large chunk of your course work, it would take sympathy from your lectures to pardon you when you are late, or absent.

The reality is that the school system is fashioned in ways that place the student at the mercy of their teachers. And as a student, you should devise means to make yourself excel even when you have particularly difficult teachers. My advice is that you try to be in the good books of your teachers but if you have done all in your power to achieve this and you know for a fact that he has bluntly refused to change his countenance towards you, I suggest you do your best and start documenting events with him so that if and when you do take the matter to the appropriate authority you will have proof to back up your accusations.

"The real winners in life are the people who look at every situation with an expectation that they can make it work or make it better"
Barbara Pletcher

Rapid Change in Medical Information:

People say the only thing constant in life is change; in medical school, you understand the implication of this first hand. Information changes at an alarming rate- yearly, a protocol for patient management are updated, in some cases, you are advised to do something totally contrary to what was previously considered to be normal. The irony is that they expect you, the medical student to be abreast of these changes.

I remember one of my lecturers saying that you don't know is not an excuse in medicine, you will be entrusted with someone's life and they definitely would not want to condone your ignorance. I believe that I have repeated several times that a bulk of what you study in medical school as a medical student would either be considered un- correct or updated when you start practicing. So you need to continue studying, and of course, properly understand all you are being taught because when the changes come you should recognize why, and easily appreciate and implement them.

What you should realize is that when you finish medical school, schooling or rightly put, learning isn't quite finished! As you start to practice you will need to continue this learning process. You will read journals, articles, textbooks, yes, textbooks! For updates and improvement in patient management and to refresh your memory on things you may have forgotten. Just think about it for a moment, having already crossed the intricate hurdle of getting into a medical school, you could only barely survive the six years of schooling only to be told when you are through that is it not over, as a matter of fact, it is only just the beginning. This is the lot of the medical student, the challenges we have to face, and the psychological, physical and spiritual hurdles we need to cross. People say what does not kill you only make you stronger, I guess in medicine we are strong because we survive the difficulties that come our way.

"I do not want to die...until I have faithfully made the most of my talent and cultivated the seed that was placed in me until the last small twig has grown"
Kathe Kollwitz

CHAPTER FIVE

THE SIX-YEAR MEDICAL SCHOOL SYSTEM

Most people know that in schools around the world, medicine is studied on average for six years. But what they may not know is that these years are not simply random, rather they are patterned in a way that information given to students structurally builds on itself. It is pretty much synonymous to building a house, as each block is laid upon another so is information dispersed in medical school. And as expected the higher you go the more difficult it becomes, however, the astute medical student is expected to fully grasp what they are taught at all levels and in the given time frame so that the outcome (the building) which in this case is their medical degree would not just be a mere paper but a testament to what they are capable of accomplishing. Contractors say that the strength of a house is all in its foundations, so it is in medicine. To be able to stand the test of time the importance of a solid foundation cannot be over emphasized. That is why you are to take every aspect of your medical study seriously.

In this chapter, we shall be dissecting the six years medical school model with the intention of revealing the rationale for its design and to give you sound principles on how you can survive your six years stay and studies as you transcend from one year to another.

It is almost certain to find that in medical schools where medicine is studied for six years, you can broadly divide these study years into two halves, the first three years consists of the pre-clinical years where students are exposed to courses categorized as the basis of medical sciences. And the next three years are usually characterized as the clinical years, as medical students are taught the fundamental principles and practice of clinical medicine and patient care.

One question I am frequently asked by students is, which segment of the above division is most important or which years should they concentrate their energy and resources? My answer always is "ALL". Yes, all the years are equally important and you should take seriously every single year of your medical study. Remember the analogy that medical school is like building a house, we can all agree that having a solid foundation is as important as erecting a good roof, no single part is greater than the other, so I want you to dismiss all the myths you may have heard about waiting until your third year or penultimate year before you become serious, since this would not help you in the six-year medical school model.

At this point, I want to discuss the separate parts of the six-year medical school division and make clear the requirements of the medical students. You should realize that a vast majority of the opinions I will be stating here are only generalized as each medical school would have a unique curriculum. But I have limited myself to establishing the precepts of this book, which is to serve as a guide. In other words, what I propose here is simply a guide to give you an understanding of what your medical school should be like, if however, you want something definitive, I suggest you consult with your school administration.

The first half- the Basic Medical science years
This refers to the first three years of your medical school. In most schools, this period is used to expose students to the basics of medical practice. Students are taught fundamental scientific principles in disciplines that mirror the background of the practice of medicine. And as such, courses that form the core or foundation of medicine are often covered during this period. They include

Human Anatomy: this is the study of structures of the human body

Human Histology: considered a subdivision of anatomy and it is the microscopic analysis of the cell structure of the human body via the use of certain contrasting agent that aid resolution and viewing

Human Embryology: Another subdivision of anatomy that discusses the detailed description of the development of structures of the human body. If you are interested in how parts of your body came into being, embryology would give you the answers.

Human Physiology: this refers to the study of the functions of different organs, systems with respect to structure.

Medical Biochemistry: here, you will be exposed to the study of how different biological and chemical agents or factors affect structures of the body and ultimately help the body to function as an orchestrated unit.

Medical Microbiology: here you do not only learn the properties of different microorganisms but you are taught how each adversely affects the health of an individual.

Pathology: which in oversimplified terms is the opposite of physiology, I try to let students understand that physiology is closely related to pathology. The truth is that if you truly understand your physiology, coming up with principles of the basis of pathology should not be much of a problem. In pathology, you consider what happens when physiology fails and you are taught all about diseases their causes, mechanisms, complications etc.

Medical Pharmacology: here you are required to utilize the principles you gathered from physiology and biochemistry to determine and understand both the effect a drug has on the body and vice versa.

Immunology: you learn how the body deals with certain pathologic states, fights infections and protect us from harmful organisms and agents that reside all around us.

Other courses that may be included in this period are subjects that perhaps have no direct concatenation to medicine when looked at on surface level. They are ethics, philosophy, psychology, medical informatics, physics, history of medicine, and medical economics. Even though these courses seem unimportant at first glance I often enjoin student to take them seriously because your teachers would often find a way to connect them to medicine. And even when they don't, it is still your responsibility to find those connections and discover how using the principles you learn from these courses would help you understand the practice of modern medicine.

At the end of the first three years, a hardworking medical student should be able to appropriately describe the human body using the right medical terms, state the function of all organs and systems, explain their linkages to one another, properly elucidate the different pathologic mechanisms and state the most appropriate medication or groups of medications used for their management.

Certainly from the above discussion you can clearly see that what you learn gradually builds on itself, and it is much interwoven. Therefore, you cannot totally understand one aspect without first understanding the previous. The classic example of this is Anatomy and Physiology; you cannot fully comprehend the functions of an organ if you don't know the components of the organs' structure. Also, you may have realized that the first three years often culminate with the learning of the mechanisms of different diseases- pathology and the drugs used in their management- Pharmacology. It is important to fully grasp the principles you learn in these areas because a bulk of what you know here will determine how much you understand in the following three years.

My advice to you is that you should not take these first three years for granted. Believe me; these years ultimately determine how your stay in medical school turn out and indeed what sort of doctor you become. If you properly managed this period and totally learn, memorize and completely understand all you are taught, you can be sure that the next three years would be much less hectic; in fact, some have described it as a walk in the park! I know a number of students who mistakenly neglect these preliminary years, believing they can make up for their lackadaisical behavior in subsequent years. But they end up paying for this dear mistake, as this places a tremendous strain on them and makes their medical journey even more difficult. Most of them had to re-read and learn these courses afresh! All because they didn't pay adequate attention the first time around, not only is their time wasted, but they most certainly also had bad grades.

In addition, you should know that a bulk of what you learn during these three years would form the basis of your medical education, interestingly, quite a number of the complaints you will hear from your patients during history taking or what is popularly called clerking can be explained if you adequately and efficiently understand the principles you are taught.

Another reason you should take these first three years seriously is because most universities require you to write an examination at their completion. And more so you are to pass this examination before moving to the next level. Since this exam signifies three years of your life, I don't want you to go thinking that you can understand everything you will be tested on the night before or two weeks prior to the exams, as most students do! Your best bet is to commence learning all your courses with the examination in mind. This would help create and master the right structure for the way you should prepare for classes and answer questions. So that when it's time for the examination, you will notice that more than half of your work is done and your preparations would not be as hectic as others!

Even after writing and passing the examination for basic medical science I usually encourage students to go over certain courses again, this time on their own. This would help them create new connections and solidify the connections already made. This reading could be in the form of reading their old lecture notes again, or some lecture material or summarized document. And this should be done especially for the following courses: Pathology, Pharmacology, and Biochemistry. As you may have noticed, these courses have pronounced and established bearings on understanding the fundamentals of clinical medicine. And as I have discovered, most students that engage in this activity find it easy to transition to clinical disciplines.

Before I tell you about the clinical years, I would like to raise a valid point here. One that has gained increased acceptance in quite a number of medical schools. You see, it is easy to be engrossed in the study of basic medical science that you forget that the sole purpose of studying medicine is to treat real patients with real problems and save lives. Therefore, many schools encourage teaching these preliminary courses from a clinical standpoint. In other words, as you learn, your Anatomy, Physiology, Pathology, Biochemistry, and other courses taught in basic medical years, you are to do so with respect to their clinical relevance. Personally, I prefer this method because it kindles the intuition of the novel medical student and gives him the feeling of being part of the medical team as they are saddled with the responsibility of making conclusions on situations that they would experience on a daily basis as they practice medicine. Undoubtedly this method also makes the transition to clinical learning much easier as the astute student can not only identify different diseases but can succinctly explain their underlying mechanisms and their untoward effect on various organs and systems.

The Second Half- The Clinical Years

The clinical years are somewhat different from the formative years in the sense that you only get to build on what you have already learnt. Just for emphasis, remember that the keywords here are **building on what you have already learnt!** This is because by this time you are expected to be aware of more than ninety percent of all the disease known to man with an idea of their possible management. And the remaining ten percent would be diseases that you would subsequently encounter as you start the different specialties of the clinical period.

The clinical years are characterized by learning different management and protocols for various diseases in the different specialties. In a way, this is where the glamor and façade of being a medical doctor starts. You are exposed to real patients and allowed to carry out simple noninvasive medical procedures, in some institutions you may be allowed to take patient history, and ultimately work as a doctors' assistant. I tell you this, from experience, if you did truly grasp what you learnt in your first three years of studying, the next three years are usually quite interesting. You will easily become the envy of your colleagues and teachers! The truth is that this is not a time where you are taught the basics of medicine- no one would have the patience to go through all those preliminary things with you anymore and you will most probably be mocked, insulted or scolded if you don't really know them.

The following are the courses you will do in the clinical years

Internal medicine: here you study diseases and their management with respect to different organs and systems, such as Cardiology, Hematology, Pulmonology, Urology, Gastroenterology, Endocrinology, Ophthalmology and others

Obstetrics and Gynecology: you are taught the diseases that are evident in women and the characteristic of the reproductive cycle of women, the process of pregnancy, labor and delivery and their different pathologic mechanisms and management.

Surgery: you will learn the indication for most surgical procedures, understand the principles of surgical managements and describe different surgical techniques. You may even be allowed to scrub in and partake in a number of surgeries, depending on your institutions' policies.

Pediatrics: deals with the care of children. Given that kids are somewhat different from adults you will learn the diseases that are unique to them and the different schemes for the management of these diseases. The risk factors and causes of disease for the pediatric patient may be different from those of the adult population. You are expected to note these differences and remember the appropriate dose of medications for managing children.

Oncology: here you are taught about different cancers, their risk factors, causes, pathogenesis, complications and probable treatment options available, be it the use of chemotherapy, surgery or radiation. In addition, you will be told about different protocol and recommendation for a host of cancers. And be introduced into several preventive measures that come handy when advising your patients.

Neurology: diseases of neurological origins are considered here and a strong knowledge of neuroscience can be useful as you embark on this course.

Rheumatology: diseases of the muscles bones and joints are covered here

Psychiatry: diseases of the mind. You will be taught about the subconscious and the conscious state, different principles or neurotic and psychotic manifestations in different disease states. You will be told about the different drugs that affect the mind, their advantages, and disadvantages.

Infectious diseases: a build up from microbiology and pathology- here you learn not only the different mechanisms that cause these disorders but the different management schemes that have been proposed for their treatment.

Like you may have rightly observed, the second part of the six years medical school system requires that you go through the various specialties that we have in medicine. This period is often intensive and you will have to apply much of what you already know as you transcend from one department to another. This is definitely not the time that you should miss classes. For some odd reason, I understand that these years fly by so fast that you are forced to wonder what happen in between. But do not be dismayed because you would have learnt a lot!

All in all, you will be excited. As a medical student, the joy of being part of the medical team can be compared to nothing! It is overwhelming and no doubt you will be blown off your feet as you see all that you have spent years studying come to life. It is the interesting and new cases that you experience firsthand that would serve as enforcement of your medical knowledge making concepts engraved in your memory. For instance, the first patient I saw with a rare condition was a small girl with osteogenesis imperfect- how could I ever forget the sight of that five-year-old with seemly huge head and a small trunk and extremities. Her thin and brittle bones that made it impossible for her to move without fracturing them coupled with her radiant blue eyes that were sharp enough to pierce the toughest of hearts, making her such a charming character to behold. But despite her condition, she had hope, her hope we could all clearly see from her captivating smile and her infallible intelligence and her love for painting. After all, she was only a small beautiful girl full of expectation! Situations like these will forever remain with you, throughout your medical practice and will not only make you curious but strive to find ways to alleviate the patients' pain.

During the clinical period, you will be expected to develop practical skills. In other words, you should be able to carry out all the activities required for physical examination of a patient. This entails a proper evaluation of all organs and systems, knowing how to percuss, palpate and auscultate when need be. As a generalization, you should at least master the examination of the respiratory, gastrointestinal, urinary neurological and cardiovascular systems. You should be able to recognize normal and pathological heart sounds and murmurs determine the borders or the heart, both relative and absolute borders and note the position of the apex beat and feel for thrills. For the lungs, you should be conversant with methods to determine topographic and comparative percussion and auscultation. Learn to pick up adventitious sounds over lungs fields and passages, determine the lower border of the lungs and note its excursion when it is filled with air. You should also know how to feel for vocal fremitus. In the gastrointestinal system, you should know how to palpate all the organs of the abdominal cavity and be able to localize masses and give a different approximate measurement for any palpated masses. These practical skills can only be truly developed if you constantly visit the clinic, observe and experiment with willing patients. Proficiency comes from your exposure to a lot of patients and having the opportunity to carry out these activities repeatedly on them.

Another way students can gain proficiency in their medical skills is to attend special holiday programs where such skills are taught. Instead of wasting valuable time during holidays, medical students can enroll in some vocational course where they are taught the principles and indeed the art of physical examination and be subsequently exposed to the challenges of patient care. This advice is particularly valuable for those studying medicine in a language that is second to theirs or perhaps don't have the opportunity to have first-hand discussions with patients or be privy to the all-important one on one contact with patients.

Most medical schools consider the final year of the six years medical school model as the practice year. This means that, at this point, learning should be carried out at the bedside of patients. Students are required and certainly encouraged to be active members of the medical team. They are forced to undergo rotations and take part in compulsory ward rounds, which avails them the opportunity to see quite a number of interesting cases. Then again it is somewhat easy for the astute medical student to be carried away. Apart from the intrigues of acting like a doctor, talking with patients and doing all those interesting things, most medical schools require their students in this year to write the final or professional examination. So as a piece of advice, try not to get cut up in the euphoria of being a doctor, do prepare for your final examinations, after all, until you pass it you would never be recognized as a true physician!

Bridging the Gap

I think you should read this part carefully because I reckon this is perhaps something you are not taught in medical school. Yes, they manage to give you information day in and out about all these wonderful subjects and courses, but no one seems to care about what you do with this information, how you get to connect the dots and make your knowledge come to life. I feel really disheartened when I ask a clinical student some basic anatomy question and they tell me that they don't know or they have forgotten, and when I ask them to tell me the mechanism of a disease and they fumble. In some ways, it only seems like students read to pass their courses and get by in school for the first three years, and then they relinquish their knowledge or totally decide to forfeit it. And in the process, make ridiculous excuses or generalizations, I have heard a few of these excuses and I intend sharing them with you. It is not uncommon to hear students say "oh, there is no Anatomy, Physiology or Biochemistry in clinical, so why should I bother studying them let alone having these courses memorized?" Or "I forgot because I was not taught well!"

This way of thinking is obviously wrong and you should not fall into this trap because students that do end up making lousy mistakes when they take on the challenges of managing patients in the clinical settings. It is mandatory to know that in clinical practice you need to bring to bear all that you have learnt from you preclinical years, as a matter of fact, you should endeavor to build on the information procured in the preclinical years like builder do on a foundation. For instance, you should know that bulk of the laboratory analysis (especially blood work) that you will order during your clinical years all stem from your knowledge in understanding of biochemical principles and the ultimate effects of biochemical events that take place in the body. It is your in-depth understanding of these concepts that would aid you in not only appropriately ordering the right tests but capable of making the correct interpretations.

Another area the gap can be bridged is the study of microbiology in preclinical years and infectious disease in clinical years. To adequately understand the mechanisms involved in how different bugs cause diseases you should understand the discrete and indeed unique characteristics of the microorganisms. By doing this, you ultimately equip yourself with the arsenal that can hamper the growth and proliferation of these harmful agents, thus making it quite easy to prescribe the most appropriate medicaments that would be beneficial to your patients.

I once read that to study the phenomenon of disease without books is like to sail an uncharted sea, while to study books without patients is not to go to sea at all. The point to take home here is that in medicine there are quite a number of courses that tend to overlap in this way and you can only make life better for yourself if and when you totally understand the information given to you as soon as they are presented, and painstakingly continue to make meaningful associations that will not only make them memorize-able but easy to utilize in the nearest future.

Also as you strive to bridge this gap, I want to introduce you to a concept in medicine, this is where you, as you study you get to play a simple game, which I call "naming the most common causes". In other words, as you run through your studies, you note and take particular interest in the most common causes of diseases, or most important risk factors or clues for different disorders. This game is advantageous because in your clinical practice you will be faced mostly with the most common causes of diseases anyways, so it becomes beneficial to start getting used to the idea even as students. The fascination thing about this game is that you may decide to know the most common cause of a disease in different groups or categories of people, such as a particular age group, sex, occupation, and others. This method, whose bearings are from epidemiology aided me in making quite a number of connections between different diseases, their risk factors, susceptible populations, mechanisms of transmission and causative agents.

The truth remains that your patients would expect you to be able to bridge the gap and make these connections effortlessly to come up with reasons for their disorders and comfortably treat them. Every human is unique and chances are that the patients you will have and their disease presentation would be dissimilar to what you have frequently seen in medical practice. In other words, you may come across patients that are not simple textbook cases! And the only reasonable way to always make the right conclusions and decisions regardless of the situation would be if you properly understood normal physiologic mechanism and principles, linking them to the most appropriate pathologic derivative before coming up with the right diagnosis and subsequent relevant therapy. If you wish to be a successful and outstanding physician this is a skill you most definitely want to master, so don't take it likely. The earlier you start, the better you will become, after all, they say practice makes perfect. Commence making meaningful connections today and watch yourself become that splendid student and indeed physician that you so longed to be!

Preparing for your final examinations

As a student, this may well be the most important examinations you will have to write in your entire lifetime. Given the importance of this examination and the nature of its difficulty, would it not be prudent if you started preparing for it well before hand? It may surprise you to know that although most students is aware of the fact that quite a lot hinges on them passing this examination, not a lot put in the sufficient effort required to make the burden of passing this exam easy. To put it in other words, my simple trick to ensuring you do brilliantly in this examination is to start the preparation on time. Quite early in your studies, you should get as many past questions and materials, churn through them as you move from one year to another. You will be amazed at how much you understand and the number of questions you can possibly answer. The advantage of doing this is that you become used to the way final examination questions are set, plus, being abreast of the information, when the time for the examination comes, it would not all seem too novel to you and you would have already seen a bulk of what you will be asked about. When I tell students to read with questions in mind they giggle and sometimes don't take me too seriously. The truth is that in the real world, you will be faced with lots and lots of questions, so it imperative to start getting used to the idea of providing answers-obviously, right answers to the questions that would be inevitably asked.

> **"If your regrets linger, if you cannot find inspiration in solitude, then you still have much to learn from the writers and poets and the cooks on becoming the artist of your own life. You can never recreate the past. But you can shape your own future."**
> **Jacqueline Duval**

What I am propagating is that you get the questions before your final year, look through them, noting those that are quite familiar and those that aren't, then take the particularly difficult questions to senior colleague or mentor, have them interpret and answer them for you, you will be amazed at how the answers you get are related to the things you are currently studying. No doubt this will not only put you ahead of your class but it will help you make those important connections.

Since most final examination requires that you pass a practical skills assessment test, I suggest that you learn and perfect these skills beforehand too. You should ensure that during your rotations before you leave a particular department or specialty, you should confident that you have mastered the techniques and methods they use for physical examination of patients. However if for any reason you discover that you couldn't do this, I advise that you either make time to immediately learn this procedure or pay to have this skills learnt from a reputable institution. Like I have previously noted, there are so many summer or holiday programs held for medical students to not only teach them these invaluable skills of patient management but also create the environment for them to have the opportunity to practice and perfect their skills. And make them more proficient.

In conclusion, I want you to carry a positive mental attitude regarding your examination. It is after all, only when you pass it that you can be made a doctor! Therefore you should strive to perform brilliantly in it, while not taking any area for granted and preparing well before the appointed time.

CHAPTER SIX

CHOOSING A MEDICAL SPECIALTY

It may sound presumptuous when I say this, but as a medical student, it is good to know the area in medicine that you would most likely love to vie into. Even though your choices are bound to change as you transcend from one department to another, it is beneficial to have a framework, something you can build on. For example, if you fancy working in the laboratory as a medical scientist or if you would rather be a clinical investigator or researcher, it is advantageous to know beforehand so you can take particular interest in the courses that are related to your area of specialization as you study. I feel compelled to share this with you, I personally watched as my preferences changed from wanting to be a pathologist, to a thoracic surgeon, to a cardiologist, to an oncologist, to pediatrician! At one point I gave up trying to make up my mind because I had this belief that I would excel in whatever field I found myself. But did I stop? Of course not! I understood that the major advantage I got from temporary assuming these professions or specialties is that I usually tried to put the extra effort when I studied them or had rotations in them. My rationale was that if I wanted to end up in those fields I had to do my best and be grounded in what I learn from my studies about them, in other words, my aim was not only to have an "A" in them but to be grounded as I studied them. So I say to you, avail yourself of the same opportunity and make the most your dreams, dream big and do all in your power to achieve those beautiful dreams of yours.

After writing and passing your final examination, it is important that you pick the most befitting specialty in medicine to settle in. in this chapter, we shall talk about the importance of picking the right specialty, how to pick the right specialty and I would do my best to make a list of all the available specialties in medicine. Hopefully, by the time I am done, you should be able to relate with one specialty on my list!

The importance of choosing the right medical specialty

It is an obvious fact that we all came into medicine for different reasons and when it comes to choosing that particular specialty, it is important to take into consideration your primary motivation for coming into medical school. You have to do this so that in the end you can attain maximum satisfaction or fulfillment.

 It would be unfair for you to spend six years in medical school and another four or more years only to end up with a specialization that you totally hate or regret. Life is too short for you to live in senseless regrets or resentment. You have to be fully and firmly committed to the path you choose, if you must achieve real success then you should realize that the zeal to do your best at all times regardless of the circumstances is stoically tied to the fact that you are involved in something that you love. I have found out that many medical students and graduates who disobey this basic principle often find themselves in specializations that they eventually loathe and disregard. They end up not giving their all, not to mention best and act ultimately mediocre. Also, their robotic attitude to their various jobs not only makes them perform below average but causes them to be prone to quite a number of mistakes. If you take a cursory look at your faculty, my guess is that you will most likely see people like these individuals described above, since they are not difficult to spot. They will be the ones to walk around like they have the whole world on their shoulder, as teachers, they are often unnecessarily mean to their students, and they are lackadaisical, as doctors, they are lousy at what they do, always ready to relinquish their posts and blame others when things go wrong or make others carry their burden for them. No doubt if they were in a different specialization, they would most definitely be happier and perhaps fared better.

We all know that being in our chosen fields makes us work harder, it is this hard work that can easily translate to progress in all we do, and as such we gain respect as good physicians. Someone once said that medicine is all about making a name for yourself as you go about treating people and curing their diseases, I cannot agree any better with this assertion. If you pick the right specialization, you will soon become prestigious and people all over the world would begin to come pay homage to you for your wonderful works.

"What a different story people would have to tell if they would adopt a definite purpose and stand by that purpose until it had time to become an all-consuming purpose".
Napoleon Hill, Laws of Success

Another important aspect to consider whilst picking a specialty in medicine is your take on financial stability. It is common knowledge that some specialties in medicine lead to better pay in comparison to others. Therefore if you happen to be the sort of person that can only be motivated by financial gains, you should endeavor to settle for these lucrative areas. The bottom line remains that, the decision you eventually make is one where you are guaranteed true happiness. If at the end of the long hard day, you cannot look yourself in the mirror and be proud of the person you have become or what you see in the mirror, then I am sorry to say that you are not in the right specialty.

Convenience is another good reason to be considered before picking the right specialization. If age is not on your side or perhaps you are female and you would love to start a family right after medical school, it would certainly be wise to then settle for specializations that do not require unnecessary long hours away from home. You should take this into consideration as you make your final decision on what you intend to do. Especially as most people in your life (including your loved ones) have already made sacrifices for you in the last six years, therefore, they would expect you to make pertinent compromises and it logical that you reciprocate their gesture.

How to pick the right specialization

Your first task really is to have an in-depth knowledge yourself. You should not settle for a specialization because it happens to be what your friends like or perhaps you heard about some supposed satisfaction or gratification that someone else gets from it. No. Instead, you need to take a good look at yourself and know exactly the type of things you like and dislike, the things you can easily swallow or condone before you take the committed step or enormous leap into a specialization.

"You were born an original. Don't die a copy."
John Maso

In like manner, you need to determine your strengths and weaknesses. It makes no sense what so ever for you to settle for a specialization that you don't have the slightest clue on what is expected of you, the challenges, obstacles and gains all seems so surreal. For instance, if you are the sort of student that has always had problems with neuroscience and personally found it difficult understanding the nature of how nerves are intricately interwoven in the body, it is futile to then pursue a specialization in neurosurgery. Indeed it would be a blatant waste of valuable time, as you will come to abhor your decision. Hence before finally taking the step, I implore you to take stock of your abilities. Personally, I would suggest that you get a plain sheath of paper and list out your abilities and the specializations that you are interested in, and then try to match a specialization with the suited ability. In the end noting the specialization you have most abilities for.

In addition, you should settle for specialties in fields in line with your specified career goals. Yes your goals, remember those goals I forced you to write down in the second chapter of this book? I want you to put them into consideration. After all, they served as the basis for your studies in the past six years. Ensure that whatever you end up with is certainly in line your goals. Do remember that your goals only serve as signposts on your journey, and being reliable guides to you already, I am indeed convinced that putting them into consideration would be more than beneficial to you. As you chose your career path, do not forget to consult with your mentors. You can bounce ideas off them and use their wealth of experience to serve as a bright light to your path. You should consider meeting with your teachers or career counselors or those in the right position to point you in the appropriate direction if you happen to be confused.

I should add here that the internet can serve as a reliable, instrumental tool as you make this decision of picking a specialty. On the internet, you will find a number of resources that can help you determine the sort of doctor you should be or the specialization that best suit your personality. The interesting fact is that in most cases, these resources are free and its takes short time to fill the questioners you will be given. Quite a number of them are accurate so if you are not sure or still confused, you may do a couple of them and compare the results you obtain. The important thing here is to use them as a guide, because the ultimate decision should be based on your strengths, abilities and what makes you happy and not merely on what you get on the internet.

A laconic list of medical specializations available today will include the following:

Pathology

Thoracic surgery

General surgery

Radiology

Physical and medical rehabilitation

Hematology

Endocrinology

Occupational disease

Plastic surgery

Nuclear medicine

Neurology

Dermatology

Anesthesiology

Allergy and immunology

Radiation oncology

Infectious disease

Nephrology

Pulmonology

Radiology

Neurosurgery

Radiology

Rheumatology

General internal medicine

Colon and rectal surgery

Gastroenterology

Medical oncology

Emergency medicine

Ophthalmology

Otolaryngology

Psychiatry

Preventive medicine

Family practice

Urology

Aerospace medicine

Pediatrics

Obstetrics and gynecology

Orthopedic surgery

Please note that although this list isn't extensive I am convinced that you would find an area that is suitable for you.

CHAPTER SEVEN

GETTING READY FOR THE WORKFORCE

We are about to get to the end of our journey together. I reckon by now, you already know the twists and turns in this trip and you are well aware of the stops and challenges you are bound to face as you embark on this quest. Therefore, at this point, we would be dealing with things you should do before we finally end this glorious trip. And I have called this, getting ready for the workforce. I should be telling you about the essential preparations you are required to make before you can be fully accommodated into the working environment. You should take this seriously as it would be bad for you to be caught unprepared. You want to be ready for the transition from being a student to becoming a doctor. Frankly speaking, it is a different ball game, with somewhat different sets of rules which we shall expunge in a little while.

Before you finish medical school, one thing you should certify is the place you wish to practice. Your postgraduate study is almost as important as your medical degree years. you should at least have a short list of possible places where you can go for your compulsory medical practice since this practice can range from one year to three depending on the part of the world where you intend doing it. By now I know you must have heard that undergoing this ordeal is a prerequisite for all medical graduates as it exposes them to the manner and indeed nature of the practice of medicine in their various countries or their areas of interest. It is during this year that you are eventually taught to make the leap from being a student to becoming a fully-fledged doctor as you are gradually encouraged to care for patients with little supervision. Also, they try to teach and introduce you to more advanced and practical ways of managing patients thus making you seem more confident in yourself and your judgments, hence the importance of knowing beforehand where you intend to do this practice. If possible, visit the hospital, have a chat with an intern or doctor and determine the things you need to bring along with you when you start. Make arrangements for accommodation, feeding, and other necessities before time because if you don't when you are ready, there may be a rush for the limited facilities.

What many students fail to understand is that getting ready for the workforce is synonymous to looking for a job. You are often required to have comprehensive curriculum vitae, one that is made up of very good references. But what do we find? Most medical students would have never held a steady job before venturing into medicine, therefore their first real job search is their internship year application. As such they have little or nothing in terms of job experience to make their curriculum vitae outstanding except the odd jobs, here and there!

A good reference can make the difference. It is good to have a top member of your faculty write a reference letter for you or your chosen mentor do the same. Remember this is a document you intend to add to your curriculum vitae, hence you want them to write something good that can help to collaborate the story you have told with your CV. And having a senior member of your faculty do that can add the needed credibility to your exploits as a medical student, also you should endeavor to get your reference letter long before you graduate from your university. As a matter of fact, I advise that you start building your CV long before your graduation. This would sensitize you to get more involved in things that would make your CV even better. For example, you may be spurred into taking part in scientific symposiums and gatherings, become a summer research assistant or attend programs where you will be awarded a certificate, all of which may be included in your curriculum vitae.

Another point to note as you prepare for the workforce is that you are not to stop studying or learning because your education continues. This is the advice I was given by my oncology lecturer. Although I only had one semester with him, he drove the point home by telling me that he has managed to teach me all that was humanly possible in the short time we spent together (I even had to borrow one of his books because I didn't fancy the textbook my school provided for the course!). Immediately after my final oncology examinations, just before I left the class, he accosted me and told me that I was a good student and he was really proud being my teacher, but as I got ready for the workforce I should know that it's only just the Beginning of my studying! Because according to him, during my first few years as an intern, I will still need to consult my books once in awhile and when I look back at what he said I can't help but totally agree with him. So I tell you same thing today. As you encounter those patients, don't forget to review their cases with the most current materials available to you. I believe the most important advantage of this attitude is that it gives you a face and an emotion to attach to those mere cases. In other words, they cease to become mere words written on a piece of paper, or a book but are transformed to real individuals with fears, hopes dreams and aspirations irrespective of how difficult their circumstances may appear.

One other thing you should know as you prepare for the workforce is that you will have co-workers or colleagues and in most cases, you will be expected to work as a team, hence, the need to learn to deal with people. You want to always have a professional working environment where people can strive to be better in all that they do. Ultimately, however, you should learn to put your patient's needs first and do all in your power within the set rules of conducts to ensure that your patients are as comfortable as possible. This could mean disagreeing with a senior college, but you should do this respectfully and never make it all about your pride or knowledge because when you do this, you will end up hurting yourself or someone else.

On a lighter note, there is nothing as appalling as seeing an intern with scruffy looking white coats and dirty shoes! Listen, when you get a place for your practice, please endeavor to go buy new laboratory/ward coats, shoes, a stethoscope, a pen light, a sphygmomanometer and other valuable things that are essential for ward rounds. You certainly don't want to look like you are ill prepared for the task ahead of you. Don't use the same laboratory coats that you used as a student. I know we all have the tendency of keeping memorabilia, but these items aren't things you should make compromises on. The presentation is everything. You are joining an elite profession, therefore you should try to act, and look and sound like your esteemed colleagues. You should strive to always be responsible. Wear clothes that make people respect you. In other words, dress like you wishes to be addressed. And know that where ever you are and whatever do, you represent doctors, so let your actions not be one that would bring disgrace or disregard to this profession. Learn to be your best at all times, because that is the life you are called into.

CHAPTER EIGHT

NOW YOU ARE A DOCTOR

At this point, I can gladly inform you that we have come to the end of our journey. I believe you are now a medical doctor and you have the prefix "Dr" or "MD" to your name. How exciting it is to know that the business of saving lives starts in earnest now and you have the golden opportunity to put to practice all you have learnt for so many years.

Taking into the considerations all the efforts you have made to get to this point, I am convinced you will make a successful doctor. Why do I say this, you may be asking yourself?

The answer is simple; you have gone through the contents of this book and certainly judiciously followed its precepts, you have created your mission statement(s) and have a comprehensive action plan, therefore you easily tackle (d) the numerous problems of medical school because you were well equipped for the challenges long before they came tumbling down your way. Also, you understand the detailed anatomy of the medical education system(s) and could therefore easily make the transition from preclinical years to clinical years by maximizing your study times so you not only got "A's" but you memorized and retained more than 90 percent of all what you learnt. Above all, you sure ended up in the right specialty, since you took ample time and efforts to ensure that you settled for not only what you are good at but also on that which brings both happiness and financial gratification to you.

Indeed you are now a doctor
I want you to take a moment and think about all the numerous examinations and tests you had to write (or will write) to get to the point of being called a doctor. Imagine the hurdles that you had to scale (or will scale). I am convinced that some will be more memorable than others! Whatever the grade or the situation, you should be proud of yourself. You are (will be) found worthy in both character and learning, hence it is fit to bestow you with the degree of MD!

No doubt you are destined for greatness, the world becomes your theater and you can direct the beautiful drama of life as a medical doctor, as you so desire. But a little bit of advice for you. Do not forget where you started from. I understand that you had (or will have) a relatively easy time studying medicine because you purchased a copy of this book, nevertheless, you should strive to be humble. The knowledge you have now should only be used to propagate good deeds, remember the Hippocratic Oath? The one you swore (or will swear) to uphold in the presence of man and God!

Try not to lose sight of the time, energy, efforts and sacrifices people made to equip you with all that was needed to make you a success. During your appointed hour of glory, let these thoughts humble you and let compassion be your foundation. Do not be the type of doctor that merely love to heal people, rather genuinely love people! Because out of your love for people would stem the undeniable bond that all patients seek from their doctor. Also, let your presence be enough to calm your patients, let it bring hope and give those under your care the willingness to fight whatever malady they may be facing.

Someone once said that after graduating from medical school, it takes about one to three years for one to fully transform from being the goofy medical student that makes lots of avoidable errors to a full-fledged confident doctor. Whether this proposition is true or not, I can't honestly say, and it is not a matter for this book. But one thing is certain, though, you have what it takes to make a fast and easy transition because you have this book. I believe you understand what is expected of you and you can smoothly integrate the principles of medicine in a practical setting. All that is needed now DOCTOR is to perfect the art!

Learn to always start with what is known and gradually work your way into the unknown. Since you happen to be the sole custodian of human life, you should recognize its value and do everything in your power with every fiber of your being to preserve its sanctity.

Another important advice you should have is that you **never forget your FAMILY**. They have already endured a lot from the moment you started this journey. And it would be only fair for you to not only recognize this but make concerted efforts to listen to their needs. Although the neglect never truly stops, it is your responsibility to find the means to strike a balance between taking care of your patients and family. Do not just be blinded by money or the chase after fame or glory to the point where you relegate spending time with your kids and family. Believe me, they are as important as your patients, if not more! Invest in them, with your time, resources, money, attention and more, so that in the end, you get to reap the fruits of your labor on both fronts.

This is just a guide book telling you how to become a doctor, now you are a doctor. And I reckon this book has served its purpose. Hopefully, in the nearest future, I will have the opportunity of writing another book to inform you of how to be a fulfilled doctor and build a reputable career as a medical practitioner.

Until then, don't stop growing and

EDUCATE YOUR MIND.

<u>ABOUT THE BOOK</u>

No doubt the journey of getting a medical degree can be both difficult and frustrating. Often enshrouded with lots of complex challenges, it makes the highly intelligent amongst us cringe and cower in despair, how much more the vast majority with average intelligence!

The Medical student's guide is a book written for: those with the intention of studying medicine, medical students, interns, dentist, doctors and indeed anyone interested in understanding the inner workings of medicine or medical education.

This book is designed specifically to answer all the questions you have about the study of medicine. And if like me you are not satisfied with the answers you are getting on the numerous problems you have on your medical journey, or you don't have a family member or relative in the medical field to direct and advise you as you travel, then this book is definitely just what you need.

From this book you will learn:

☐ *About the important things, you should know before starting the journey to becoming a doctor and the basic pre-requites that are needed to be successful.*

☐ *Discover the compulsory hurdles that every medical student encounters and get tried and tested ways to cross every hurdle without much hassle*

☐ *How to transition effortlessly from preclinical to clinical years of medical school*

☐   *How to choose a befitting specialty in medicine that will make you both happy and financially gratified*

☐   *And lots more...*

You can buy this book for your child, spouse, sibling, friend or colleague that harbors the intention of going into the medical field or someone that may be currently struggling with their medical journey and watch them drastically transform!

ABOUT THE AUTHOR

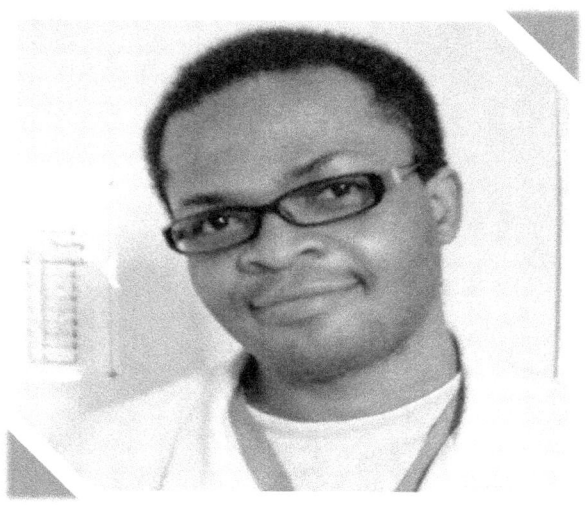

HENRY *EGBUCHIEM* is an intelligent young man who has a B.sc (human Anatomy) and an MD degree. Having spent many years in the medical field; teaching, mentoring and encouraging students, he has acquired quite a number of skills and methods to not only help his students academically but also spur them into becoming better doctors, all these secrets he has succinctly written in this book to equally inspire you.

www.ingramcontent.com/pod-product-compliance
Lightning Source LLC
Chambersburg PA
CBHW071436180526
45170CB00001B/362